Convers...

Complementary
and Alternative
Medicine

*Insights and Perspectives
from Leading Practitioners*

Norma G. Cuellar, DSN, RN, CCRN
Assistant Professor
University of Pennsylvania
School of Nursing
Philadelphia, PA

JONES AND BARTLETT PUBLISHERS
Sudbury, Massachusetts
BOSTON   TORONTO   LONDON   SINGAPORE

World Headquarters
Jones and Bartlett Publishers
40 Tall Pine Drive
Sudbury, MA 01776
978-443-5000
info@jbpub.com
www.jbpub.com

Jones and Bartlett Publishers
Canada
6339 Ormindale Way
Mississauga, Ontario
L5V 1J2
CANADA

Jones and Bartlett Publishers
International
Barb House, Barb Mews
London W6 7PA
UK

Jones and Bartlett's books and products are available through most bookstores and online book-sellers. To contact Jones and Bartlett Publishers directly, call 800-832-0034, fax 978-443-8000, or visit our website www.jbpub.com. Substantial discounts on bulk quantities of Jones and Bartlett's publications are available to corporations, professional associations, and other qualified organizations. For details and specific discount information, contact the special sales department at Jones and Bartlett via the above contact information or send an email to specialsales@jbpub.com.

ISBN-13: 978-0-7637-3888-4
ISBN-10: 0-7637-3888-3

Library of Congress Cataloging-in-Publication Data
Conversations in complementary and alternative medicine / edited by
    Norma G. Cuellar.
      p. cm.
    Includes bibliographical references and index.
    ISBN 0-7637-3888-3 (alk. paper)
    1. Alternative medicine. 2. Physicians--Interviews.   I. Cuellar,
    Norma G.
    R733.C666 2006
    610--dc22

                                        2006003529

6048

Production Credits
Executive Editor: David Cella
Production Director: Amy Rose
Production Assistant: Rachel Rossi
Editorial Assistant: Lisa Gordon
Associate Marketing Manager: Laura Kavigian
Manufacturing Buyer: Therese Connell
Composition: Jason Miranda, Spoke & Wheel
Cover Design: Timothy Dziewit
Printing and Binding: Malloy, Inc.
Cover Printing: Malloy, Inc.

Printed in the United States of America
10 09 08 07 06   10 9 8 7 6 5 4 3 2 1

Dedication

To my parents

Maria Tereza Aguilar Cuellar (1933–1996) who died of lung cancer before her time (she never smoked a day in her life). She always had faith in me and believed I could do anything if I set my mind on it, encouraging me even when I didn't believe in myself. I know she would be proud of my accomplishments and I am grateful for the time I had with her.

Ruben Dario Cuellar—is older now. But still encourages me and supports me in every way he is capable. He is one of the kindest men you will ever know—and I am grateful for this personal characteristic that he has shared with his family and so many people in our hometown of Petal, Mississippi.

To the Victims of Hurricane Katrina

My heart remains attached to my home in Mississippi where so many of my friends and family were devastated by Katrina in August 2005. Many of the modalities mentioned in this book may help provide relief of the physical and emotional trauma as a result of Katrina. My beautiful "Magnolia State" may never be the same but because of the faith of these great Southern people, they will be stronger and better for everything they have been through.

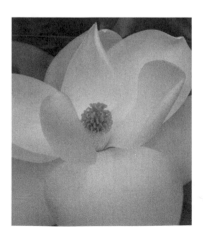

CONTENTS

PREFACE

Complementary and Alternative Medicine (CAM) research has made monumental advances in the last 10 years. Due to their rigorous research effort and commitment, CAM practitioners have persevered, maintaining professionalism and often overcoming ridicule with the intent to help patients when, often, nothing in the "Western" medical field has worked to improve health outcomes.

As a researcher and practitioner of CAM, I am often asked to do both professional and community presentations on the topic. Many questions are often asked of me. Many times, the same questions. The healthcare providers and consumers of health care often have these basic questions, which could easily be answered if they could find a practitioner that they trusted enough to ask.

This got me to thinking, what if readers had the opportunity to have an interaction with a practitioner of some of the most often used CAM modalities? If healthcare providers and patients had anything they could ask experts in CAM, what would they ask and how would they be answered? There are numerous books available about all areas of CAM, but this book is unique in the fact that it is an "interview," or a conversation, with expert leaders in the field who have both practiced and done research in their individual CAM specialties.

These experts were asked "What are the most often asked questions that you answer?" Their dynamic responses provided the chapters of this book. These chapters are presented in question and answer format. While some of the questions were standardized across practices, others were included based on the practitioners' expertise in teaching patients who use CAM.

I am so fortunate to have some of the best internationally known CAM authorities, many of whom have published and presented across the globe, as contributing authors to this book. They have been publicly recognized for their experience in their areas of practice. They have served on national and international committees to advance the science of CAM. They are leaders in professional organizations promoting health policy and the importance of choice in using CAM.

Despite their busy schedules, they also very willingly agreed to be contributing authors of this book. As you read their chapters you will hear their passion, and see just how they are changing both the practice and the perception of Complementary and Alternative Medicine by promoting research and advancing evidence-based CAM practice.

This book makes an important contribution to CAM literature because it looks at the clinician who is practicing and presents some of the driving forces that have led and directed these professionals to where they are now. It can be an inspiration to others who wonder *how* to get started and *what* needs to be done to begin a career in CAM. It gives the reader a chance to understand the educational process behind many of these modalities. It provides resources for current information as well as a historical perspective on how some of the modalities began.

This book provides the reader with resources needed to find out more about CAM modalities. It also provides information and direction for interested readers to find mentors in the areas of clinical practice, clinical professional organizations, and research.

It can serve as a supplemental text to support a course in CAM or Integrative Medicine.

ACKNOWLEDGMENTS

I want to thank all of the contributing authors for their patience and their commitment. They came from across the world to generously share with the reader first-hand insight into their individual practices.

I want to thank Jones and Bartlett for completing this project with me, and for seeing how important this book may be to many healthcare providers who still wonder what CAM is and what type of people really practice CAM.

But the most important person I want to acknowledge is my son, Matthew. I would not be where I am today if it was not for him. I strive to make him proud of me and to be a role model for him. Thank you . . . I am so very proud of the young man you are becoming . . . I love you.

CONTRIBUTORS

John Alton, BA, MFA
President, Unified Fitness, LLC
Clinical Researcher-Practitioner
Associate Faculty
Center for the Study of Complementary
  and Alternative Therapies
University of Virginia
Charlottesville, Virginia

William A. Berno, AP
Diplomate, National Board of
  Homeopathic Examiners
Private Practice
Sarasota and Clearwater, Florida

Norma G. Cuellar, DSN, RN, CCRN
Assistant Professor
School of Nursing
University of Pennsylvania
Philadelphia, Pennsylvania

Edzard Ernst, PhD, MD, FRCP (Edin.)
Director, Complementary Medicine
Peninsula Medical School
Exeter, Devon
England

James J. Fletcher, PhD
Professor Emeritus
George Mason University
Fairfax, Virginia

Lyn Freeman, PhD
President, Mind Matters Research
Anchorage, Alaska
Chair, Integrative Health Studies
Saybrook Graduate School
San Francisco, California

Daniel I. Galper, PhD
Senior Research Associate
University of Texas Southwestern
  Medical Center
Dallas, Texas

H. Lea Barbato Gaydos, PhD, RN, CNS,
  AHN-BC
Associate Professor
University of Colorado and Beth-El
  College of Nursing and Health Sciences
Colorado Springs, Colorado

Virginia Hisghman, PhD(c), AP, LAc,
  MSOM
Department of OB/GYN
University of Virginia
Charlottesville, Virginia

Kevin Kunz, BA
Reflexology Research Project
Albuequerque, New Mexico

Vasant Lad, MASc
Founder and Director, Ayurvedic Institute
Albuquerque, New Mexico

G. Frank Lawlis, PhD
Curriculum Director of Learning
Information Technologies
Principal Content Advisor to the
Dr. Phil Show
Sanger, Texas

Dana J. Lawrence, FICC, DC
Associate Professor
Palmer College of Chiropractic
Davenport, Iowa

Robert Leckridge, MBBCh, FFHom
Past-President, Faculty of Homeopathy
Glasgow Homoeopathic Hospital
Glasgow, Scotland

Kathleen A. Lipinski, RN, MSN
Private Practice
Continuing Education Coordinator &
  Teacher International Center for Reiki
  Training
President, Long Island Reiki Connection
Nesconset, New York

Patrick Miederhoff, PhD, PharmD
Professor Emeritus
School of Pharmacy
Virginia Commonwealth University
Richmond, Virginia
Director of Alternative Medicine
Patient First
Glen Allen, Virginia

Cynthia A. Parkman, RN, MSN,
  PHN, MA
Assistant Professor
California State University at Sacramento
Sacramento, California

David Reilly, FRCP, MRCGP, FFHom
Centre for Integrative Care
Director, Glasgow Homoeopathic
  Hospital
Glasgow Scotland

Marilyn J. Schlitz, PhD
Senior Scientist
California Pacific Medical Center
San Francisco, California
Vice President for Research and
  Education
Institute of Noetic Sciences
Petaluma, California

Heather A. Schmidt, PhD, DM, MA
Executive Director
Optimal Performance Institute
Dallas, Texas

Mary Cipriano Silva, RN, FAAN
Professor Emerita
College of Nursing and Health Science
George Mason University
Fairfax, Virginia
Clinical Professor
School of Public Health and Health
  Sciences
University of Massachusetts at Amherst
Amherst, Massachusetts

Victoria E. Slater, PhD, RN, AHN-BC
Private Holistic Nursing Practice
Clarksville, Tennessee

Patricia Smyth, DSN, RN, FNP-C
Associate Professor
Director Graduate Nursing Program
Western Carolina University
Chandler, North Carolina

Audrey E. Snyder, PhD(c), RN, MSN,
  ACNP-CS
Certified Massage Therapist
Assistant Professor
School of Nursing
University of Virginia
Charlottesville, Virginia

Matthew J. Taylor, PhD, PT, RYT
California Institute of Integral Studies
San Francisco, California
Director, Dynamic Systems
  Rehabilitation, PLLC
Scottsdale, Arizona

Michael Traub, ND, DHANP, CCH
Director, Lokahi Health Center
Kailua Kona, Hawaii

James C. Whorton, PhD
Professor
School of Medicine
University of Washington
Seattle, Washington

1

History of Complementary and Alternative Medicine

James C. Whorton, PhD

About the Author

James C. Whorton is a professor in the Department of Medical History and Ethics at the University of Washington School of Medicine. He holds a BS in Chemistry from Duke University (1964) and a doctorate in History of Science from the University of Wisconsin (1969). Dr. Whorton teaches courses on the history of medicine, history of public health, history of health beliefs and behavior, and on alternative and complementary medicine. He has published articles in all these areas in journals such as *Bulletin of the History of Medicine, Journal of the History of Medicine and Allied Sciences, Pharmacy in History, Journal of Sport History*, and *Journal of the American Medical Association*. In addition, he has published four books: *Nature Cures: The History of Alternative Medicine in America* (Oxford University Press, 2002), which has just been released in paperback; *Inner Hygiene: Constipation and the Pursuit of Health in Modern Society* (Oxford University Press, 2000); *Crusaders for Fitness: The History of American Health Reformers* (Princeton University Press, 1982); and *Before Silent Spring: Pesticides and Public Health in Pre-DDT America* (Princeton University Press, 1974).

Q: What got you interested in the history of Complementary and Alternative Medicine (CAM)?

A: I'm a historian of medicine and became aware of CAM when I began reading medical literature from the early 1800s. I was struck by how frequently physicians of the time complained about something they called "irregular medicine." As I continued to read, I realized that irregular medicine was simply the original term for what we are now calling CAM: therapies not generally employed or recognized by the mainstream medical profession. Then as I delved deeper into 19th-century irregular medicine, I came to appreciate that awareness of these historical antecedents was essential to understanding CAM today. I have subsequently written a book exploring the history of CAM as a means of shedding light on contemporary questions relating to unconventional medical practices.[1]

Q: How long has CAM been around?

A: CAM first appeared in the late 1700s. There had been plenty of dissent and differing opinions about proper treatments in medicine before that time, but dissatisfaction with orthodox medicine had not previously taken the form of organized systems of care. These new systems enlisted large numbers of practitioners who all administered the same therapies, adhered to the same theory, and proclaimed the superiority of their methods and beliefs to those of the majority profession.

Q: How is CAM different from folk medicine?

A: Folk medicine consists largely of plant and animal remedies and physical procedures intermixed with superstition and magic (e.g., a particular drug should be taken during a full moon or only after reciting a certain spell). Folk healers are generally unschooled, learning their methods through oral traditions passed from generation to generation, and practice as individuals instead of organizing into professional groups. CAM practitioners historically have discovered their own distinctive therapies through experience and then incorporated them into theoretical frameworks that draw on contemporary scientific ideas. Furthermore, they attempt to recruit new practitioners to their system and organize professionally. By the mid-1800s, most CAM systems had established schools to train new practitioners, begun publishing journals, and organized local, state, and even national societies.

Q: Why did CAM appear when it did?

A: CAM emerged partly as a reaction to the confusion that characterized 18th-century "regular" medicine, that was beset by a proliferation of erroneous theories of pathology formulated to make sense of all the new information that had been uncovered in anatomy, physiology, and chemistry during the 1600s and 1700s. CAM developers sought to establish systems of treatment based on experience with patients and common sense instead of being deduced from rational theory. They were also rebelling against the standard therapies derived from theory, treatments that included bleeding, purging the intestinal tract, and blistering the skin; CAM was a call for gentler methods that supported the efforts of nature to heal the body. Finally, CAM appeared in response to the trend of medicine to focus on the pathology of disease instead of on the patient affected by the disease. From the beginning, CAM practitioners were preaching what eventually, in the 1970s, came to be called holistic medicine, treatment of the whole patient.

Q: **Was it only these medical considerations that inspired the development of CAM, or were other factors involved?**

A: CAM was also a political movement, sparked by the enactment during the early 1800s of state laws that required medical practitioners to be licensed. These licensing laws allowed only regular physicians to practice. They were regarded by irregulars as undemocratic because they granted a medical monopoly to an elite group purely on the basis of education and prevented healers who believed in unconventional therapies from pursuing the calling of their choice, denying citizens the freedom to select whatever form of care they preferred. During the 1830s and 1840s, irregular doctors campaigned for the repeal of licensing laws and succeeded in having them removed from the statute books of virtually every state in the country.

Q: **How would you compare the popularity of CAM in former centuries with their popularity today?**

A: From the mid-1800s to the mid-1900s, CAM was roughly as popular as today. Surveys done in the 1920s, for example, indicated that a third or more of Americans were patronizing CAM practitioners at that time. The public became much more deeply impressed with the power of orthodox medicine after the appearance of sulfa drugs in the 1930s and antibiotics in the 1940s. They strayed away from CAM until the 1970s, when alternative medicine began to regain popular support.

Q: **What were the most popular CAM systems in the early days, and who were the founders?**

A: Most popular of all was homeopathy, developed in the late 1700s by the German physician Samuel Hahnemann. Homeopathy, meaning "like the disease," treated illness with extremely small doses of drugs that duplicated the symptoms experienced by the patient ("like cures like" was its operating assumption); it became established in the United States in the 1830s (see Chapter 8). Also widely accepted in America in the first half of the 1800s was Thomsonianism, a program of healing with botanical remedies developed by New Hampshire farmer Samuel Thomson. Mesmerism, or hypnosis, stemmed from the work of Viennese physician Franz Anton Mesmer in the later 1700s and came to America in the 1830s (see Chapter 11).

Finally, there was hydropathy, a system of treating disease with baths and other applications of cold water formulated by Austrian farmer Vincent Priessnitz in the 1820s; it gained a foothold in America in the 1840s.

Q: Did any new CAM appear after the first half of the 19th-century?

A: Yes. Osteopathy, which treated all disease through musculo-skeletal manipulation, was developed in the 1870s by Andrew Still.[2] In the 1890s, two other CAM appeared: chiropractic, a system of skeletal manipulations different from those of osteopathy, discovered by Daniel David Palmer (see Chapter 16), and naturopathy, an approach to treatment that used natural substances and agencies to stimulate the body to heal itself, founded by Benedict Lust (see Chapter 9).[3,4] In addition, spiritual and mental healing methods flourished in the late 1800s, most notably Christian Science, introduced in the 1870s by Mary Baker Eddy.

Q: How did orthodox medicine react to the development of CAM?

A: Regular physicians regarded CAM as unscientific, ineffective, and potentially dangerous therapies that exploited the ignorance and gullibility of the public. A 19th-century physician offering his opinion of homeopathy expressed typical feelings. Homeopathy, he stated, "should be considered the unclean thing—foul to the touch, wicked and treacherous to the soul, the death of every upright principle"; the only attitudes to have toward it were those of "abomination, loathing and hate." Acting on those attitudes, the regular profession censured members who had any professional dealings with irregulars and successfully opposed the appointment of CAM practitioners to positions in public hospitals, medical schools, and the military medical corps. In the 20th-century, MDs fought hard to keep individual states from passing licensing laws for irregulars.

Q: Where did the term "allopathic medicine" come from and what does it mean?

A: "Allopathy" was coined by Samuel Hahnemann, the founder of homeopathy, to designate regular medicine.[5] The word is derived from Greek roots meaning "other than the disease," and was meant to convey that conventional medicine did not follow homeopathy's rule of "like cures like," but sought instead to overpower disease with remedies opposite to patients' symptoms. By the mid-1800s, allopathy and allopathic medicine had been adopted by all CAM practitioners as derogatory labels for orthodox practice and were terms much resented by MDs. "Allopathic medicine" faded from use during the mid-1900s, but has been brought back in recent years, and this time without significant protest from mainstream physicians.

Q: What terms have been used historically to identify CAM?

A: The original term "irregular medicine" was most common up to the early 20th-century, but then yielded to "medical cultism" and "medical sectarianism," characterizations intended to suggest CAM was more a form of religious fanaticism than medical science. "Cultism" remained popular into the 1970s, but then steadily gave way to "alternative medicine" when CAM began to make a comeback. By the 1980s, "complementary medicine" was being used in the United Kingdom, but did not gain a footing in America until the mid-1990s when it was quickly transformed into the acronym CAM, for Complementary and Alternative Medicine. Subsequently, "integrative medicine," with its suggestion that all healing modalities can be brought together into a single grand system, has gained favor.

Q: When did licensure begin for CAM?

A: Medical licensure for CAM practitioners began in the late 1800s. At that point, the germ theory had transformed surgery and public health and allopathic medicine was enjoying much greater public respect than earlier in the century. In that atmosphere, MDs were able to get licensing laws reinstituted, and rather than oppose such laws as they had in the early 1800s, irregular doctors now demanded their own licensing protection. Homeopaths and osteopaths both succeeded in a few states by 1900, and by 1920 the same could be said for chiropractors and naturopaths. Osteopathy and chiropractic would continue to win licensing protection; by the mid-1970s, both systems would be licensed in every state. Naturopathic medicine is now licensed in thirteen states.

Q: Have there been other forms of societal endorsement of CAM?

A: Yes. For example, coverage of osteopathic medical services was included in the Medicare system established in 1965, and osteopaths were granted the right to medical appointments in the military the following year. Chiropractic was brought into Medicare in 1974. Most significant was the founding of an Office of Alternative Medicine at the National Institutes of Health through action of the Senate in 1991, an office that was upgraded to the National Center for Complementary and Alternative Medicine in 1998. And in 2000, a White House Commission on Complementary and Alternative Medicine Policy was appointed by President Clinton.

Q: When did CAM associate with Asian healing traditions in the United States?

A: In the early 1970s, the use of acupuncture as a surgical anesthetic by Chinese physicians was observed by visiting American doctors. Fascination with acupuncture quickly expanded into interest in Asian healing methods of all varieties, most particularly Chinese herbal medicine, Ayurveda, and shiatsu.

Q: Are there any similarities or shared emphases between the many forms of CAM?

A: Although each CAM system has its own distinctive therapies and theories, all share a common philosophy, a set of values that has characterized unorthodox medicine from the outset. All claim to employ natural healing, in the sense of using treatments that support and stimulate the body's own innate healing power. In addition, all profess holistic practice, treating the mental, emotional, and spiritual elements of illness as well as the physical components of disease. Finally, all maintain that practice must be rooted in clinical experience, not rationally derived from scientific theory. Indeed, some CAM groups (e.g., homeopathy) have no clear theoretical explanation for the efficacy of their methods, but are not bothered by that since they are certain from experience that their therapies work.

Q: Have allopathic physicians altered their attitudes toward CAM?

A: The disdain that allopaths have felt for CAM historically has been softening since the 1970s. Mainstream medicine has itself embraced a holistic orientation that makes it more receptive to alternative medical philosophy. Further, as physicians have become aware that more and more patients are seeking help from CAM practitioners, they have been forced to become better acquainted with unconventional healers and have found them to be better educated and more professional than had been expected. The result has been a new degree of tolerance toward CAM providers, and though much skepticism remains, cooperation between MDs and CAM doctors has expanded markedly over the last two decades, evidenced by increased referrals to unconventional practitioners, the extension of HMO coverage to chiropractic, acupuncture, and other alternative services, and even the opening of natural medicine clinics where allopaths work side-by-side with naturopaths and other CAM practitioners.

Q: Have there been any changes in the attitudes of CAM practitioners toward allopathic medicine? Why?

A: For much of the past 200 years, unconventional healers were as dismissive of allopathic medicine as it was of them, and hoped one day to see it destroyed and their own system (whichever one it might be) rule triumphant as the only form of medicine. By the mid-1900s, though, mainstream medicine was demonstrating such extraordinary powers in surgery and the treatment of infectious disease that CAM doctors could no longer plausibly condemn it as useless. Nor could they any longer imagine that their own methods were cure-alls. In recent decades, a rapprochement has been reached, in which allopathic medicine has come to be recognized as superior in the treatment of trauma and acute infection, while CAM practitioners regard themselves as better at dealing with many chronic conditions. In this environment, both sides are open to working with one another in ways that could not have been envisioned 50 years ago.[6,7]

Q: Doesn't CAM work simply through the placebo effect?

A: From the beginning, allopathic commentators have attributed the recovery of CAM patients to the action of the placebo effect and the power of the body to restore itself to health in most instances no matter what treatment it receives. As a 19th-century MD said of homeopathy, it would work every bit as well "were the similars left out and atoms of taffy or sawdust substituted, to give their patients room to exercise their faith, and nature time and opportunity to do the work." Such sentiments are still often expressed to explain the success of CAM practices, but more and more allopathic physicians are acknowledging that there may well be positive physiological actions beyond placebo effect. Clinical trials supporting the efficacy of chiropractic manipulations, naturopathic herbs, acupuncture treatments, homeopathic remedies, and other CAM therapies are suggesting that there are indeed valuable methods under the CAM heading. By the same token, it is likely that at least some, and conceivably many, CAM treatments will be found not to stand up to rigorous clinical testing. Careful and thorough research on CAM is in the beginning stages and it will be some time before it is clear which therapies are simply placebo and which are something more.[8]

Q: Has CAM brought about any changes in allopathic medical practice?

A: As the CAM emphasis on holistic medicine has gained an airing, it has worked (along with movements developing within allopathic medicine) to make MDs more attuned to the influence of mind and emotions on health, and more sensitive to the patient's subjective experience of illness and need to be treated as a unique human being instead of a case of a particular disease. Similarly, the CAM stress on cooperating with nature in the healing process has influenced physicians to be less aggressive in attacking disease with pharmaceuticals.

Q: Is CAM a passing fad, or is it here to stay?

A: Historians are not, as a rule, reliable fortune-tellers, but it seems unlikely for the foreseeable future that mainstream medicine will find cures for all diseases. There will continue to be patients whose ailments are not removable by conventional methods, or who individually do not respond well even to effective allopathic therapies, and so turn to other systems of care. This will be true even if the major CAM groups should achieve integration into the establishment and cease to be independent alternatives. New outside groups, new CAM, may thus appear to meet the needs of those patients who fail to find satisfaction with any of the therapies of an integrative medicine that has absorbed the old CAM.

References

1. Whorton JC. *Nature Cures: The History of Alternative Medicine in America.* New York: Oxford University Press; 2002.

2. Osborn GG. Taking osteopathic distinctiveness seriously: historical and philosophical perspectives. [comment]. *Journal of the American Osteopathic Association.* May 2005;105(5):241–244.

3. Meeker WC, Haldeman S. Chiropractic: a profession at the crossroads of mainstream and alternative medicine. [see comment]. *Annals of Internal Medicine.* Feb 5 2002;136(3):216–227.

4. McCabe P. Naturopathy, Nightingale, and nature cure: a convergence of interests. *Complementary Therapies in Nursing & Midwifery.* Feb 2000;6(1):4–8.

5. Jonas WB, Kaptchuk TJ, Linde K. A critical overview of homeopathy. [see comment]. *Annals of Internal Medicine.* Mar 4 2003;138(5):393-399.

6. Milden SP, Stokols D. Physicians' attitudes and practices regarding complementary and alternative medicine. *Behavioral Medicine.* 2004;30(2):7382.

7. Greenfield SM, Innes MA, Allan TF, Wearn AM. First year medical students' perceptions and use of complementary and alternative medicine. *Complementary Therapies in Medicine.* Mar 2002;10(1):27–32.

8. Kaptchuk TJ. The placebo effect in alternative medicine: can the performance of a healing ritual have clinical significance? *Annals of Internal Medicine.* Jun 4 2002;136(11):817–825.

Health Information, Managed Care, and Complementary and Alternative Medicine

Cynthia A. Parkman, RN, MSN, PHN, MA

About the Author

Cynthia A. Parkman is an assistant professor in nursing leadership and management as well as case management at California State University in Sacramento. She has recently studied women's preferences for CAM and conventional healthcare services, and studied inclusion of CAM into nursing school curricula in the United States. Among previous various publications, she writes a feature column on CAM in *The Case Manager*, the *Journal of the Case Management Society of America*. She is currently working on her PhD in sociology with an emphasis on the history of medical practice and women's healthcare in medical sociology at the University of California, Davis.

Q: What is CAM?

A: Most Americans are familiar with complementary terms used in health care today and may have read about these treatments in articles in newspapers, women's journals, and other media. Most adults are using some form of complementary or alternative medicine (CAM) or complementary and alternative therapies. To understand where current terms have come from, it is helpful to compare complementary care from alternative health care. Generally, alternative medicine is defined as any type of treatments or therapies used in place of, or instead of, conventional medicine (also known as Western medicine or allopathy). An example of an alternative therapy is using a special diet to treat cancer instead of undergoing surgery, radiation, or chemotherapy that has been recommended by a conventional doctor. Complementary medicine involves use of alternative therapies together with conventional medicine. An example of a complementary therapy is using aromatherapy to help lessen a patient's discomfort following surgery. A third category called integrative medicine combines conventional medical treatments with CAM that have been studied and determined to be safe and effective for use in health care. In addition, integrative medicine now is focusing more on holistic health care that involves the whole person, not just treatments for illnesses.

Q: What are the types of treatments classified as CAM?

A: In the past, many experts have realized that much of what conventional medicine professionals thought was complementary care is not seen that way by consumers. For example, when surveys have been done on use of CAM, many people have not listed chiropractic as an alternative therapy as they are covered by their insurance or a practitioner they have visited for years. Also, many cultures use therapies that are new to the United States but are part of various cultures' background from their own country. However, for simple classifying of CAM, is it helpful to use the current National Institution of Healthcare (NIH), National Center for Complementary Alternative Medicine definitions on the many types of CAM available in the world. **Table 2.1** lists and describes these categories of CAM.

Q: Why do people choose to use CAM?

A: CAM is far different than conventional medical therapies in fundamental areas. While conventional medicine focuses on illness (caused by an organism that invades the unsuspecting host) and interventions to reverse the deteriorative physiological process of disease, CAM focuses on wellness and the belief that the mind and body are integrated (holism). CAM is grounded in maximizing one's potential, harmony, and balance of energy.

Table 2.1   National Center for Complementary and Alternative Medicine (NCCAM) Classifications

Alternative Medical Systems	Alternative medical systems are built upon complete systems of theory and practice. Often, these systems have evolved apart from and earlier than the conventional medical approach used in the United States. Examples of alternative medical systems that have developed in Western cultures include homeopathic medicine and naturopathic medicine. Examples of systems that have developed in non-Western cultures include traditional Chinese medicine and Ayurveda.
Mind-Body Interventions	Mind-body interventions use a variety of techniques designed to enhance the mind's capacity to affect bodily function and symptoms. Some techniques considered CAM in the past have become mainstream (e.g., patient support groups, biofeedback, and cognitive-behavioral therapy). Other mind-body techniques are still considered CAM, including hypnosis, yoga, meditation, prayer, mental healing, and therapies that use creative outlets such as art, music, or dance.
Biologically-Based Therapies	Biologically-based therapies in CAM use substances found in nature, such as herbs, foods, and vitamins. Some examples include dietary supplements, herbal products, and the use of other so-called "natural," but as yet scientifically unproven therapies (e.g., using shark cartilage to treat cancer).
Manipulative and Body-Based Methods	Manipulative and body-based methods in CAM are based on manipulation and/or movement of one or more parts of the body. Some examples include chiropractic or osteopathic manipulation, and massage.
Energy Therapies	Energy therapies involve the use of energy fields. They are of two types: • Biofield therapies are intended to affect energy fields that allegedly surround and penetrate the human body. The existence of such fields has not yet been scientifically proven. Some forms of energy therapy manipulate biofields by applying pressure and/or manipulating the body by placing the hands in, or through, these fields. Examples include Qi Gong, Reiki, and Therapeutic Touch. • Bioelectromagnetic-based therapies involve the unconventional use of electromagnetic fields, such as pulsed fields, magnetic fields, or alternating current or direct current fields.

Q: What is the purpose of CAM?

A: Throughout the world, CAM plays a central role in maintaining health and treating disease. Many cultures use "traditional" therapies as part of normal life, therapies that Americans consider to be alternative. Chinese herbal therapy, a common feature in China and much of the Chinese-American community, has often been considered a type of alternative therapy in the United States. Ayurvedic medicine, with its roots in India, has begun to take hold in the United States as a form of complementary therapy, yet it is a common healthcare practice in its country of origin. Several trends that have spurred this movement and will continue to increase the demand for CAM choices include

- aging of the population with an increased concern for holistic "balanced" options for health maintenance and managing chronic health conditions;
- Baby Boomers' demands for self-care information and strategies; the high cost of both physical and mental health care; dismay over the limitations of many managed care plans; further integration of other cultural practices into conventional medical arenas, such as acupuncture, Ayurvedic medicine, etc.; and,
- increased access to information on CAM therapies—mass media, the World Wide Web, advertisements, and word-of-mouth reports.

Q: What are the pros and cons of CAM use?

A: According to Ebrahim Samba, World Health Organization (WHO) Regional Director for Africa, the widespread use of CAM makes it extremely important to evaluate its safety, efficacy, quality, and standardization. Work on national policy addressing use of CAM has been underway for many years. At the personal level, there must be careful consideration of the safety and purpose of a particular CAM. For example, although herbal products are widely available, they may have harmful side effects or untoward effects when combined with prescription drugs.

In addition, most CAM are paid for out-of-pocket and may be quite expensive when compared to a given conventional therapy that is covered by an insurance plan. An informed consumer will have the most success in navigating many sources of information on CAM and making the most educated choices among therapies considered.

Q: Compared to conventional medicine, what is the efficacy and cost of CAM use?

A: The issue of comparing costs of conventional medicine to CAM is difficult for many reasons. While conventional clinical office costs may seem low for patients with insurance with low payments for office visits, the actual cost is much higher and paid by the insurance company. Also, pharmacy costs for many people with ongoing medical needs have become a large part of their monthly budgets. A visit to a CAM practitioner may seem costly when paying out of pocket (such as $65 for a 1-hour massage, or $100 for an acupuncture visit), but if the individual can reduce drug needs and handle chronic illness symptoms well with CAM, there may be less cost for future health needs.[1] Current NIH research is paying attention to cost, efficacy, and access while comparing CAM to conventional medicine costs.

Q: What are the trends in insurance coverage of CAM?

A: Although first trends in the late 1990s were promising, there is a long road to travel before CAM are covered by a majority of insurance companies. Insurance companies are paying close attention to the billions of dollars exchanging hands in the CAM therapy world. According to surveys done from 1997 to the present, many managed care plans—in response to the public's growing interest—offer benefits for chiropractic, acupuncture, and massage therapy. Many insurance companies have already begun to integrate CAM with conventional medical providers. Some offer benefits for hypnotherapy, biofeedback, acupressure, and reflexology. See the following caveat about the reality of insurance coverage.

Q: How does managed care influence the use of CAM?

A: While most people pay for CAM therapies out-of-pocket, many say the availability of alternative therapy is important in choosing a health plan. The CAM or integrative medicine market is growing fast and consumers are driving many HMOs to consider coverage. In spite of this close attention, not all HMOs have fully embraced the concept of routine reimbursement for CAM care, and that is a key concern in the future of integrative medicine.

Q: Why do some insurance plans cover CAM (such as chiropractic, massage, or acupuncture) and others do not?

A: Few CAM therapies are covered by insurance and the amount of coverage offered varies depending upon the insurer and the state. Before agreeing to a treatment that a CAM practitioner suggests, you should check with your insurer to see if they will cover any portion of the therapy's cost. If insurance does cover a portion of the cost, you will want to ask if the practitioner accepts your insurance or participates in your insurer's network. Even with insurance, you may be responsible for a percentage of the cost of therapy.

Q: Are there any drawbacks to insurance coverage of CAM?

A: From the consumers' viewpoint, one of the first things they worry about when they hear insurance companies may cover CAM is what will happen to their access to herbal supplements. Although herbal products are not regulated in the way conventional drugs are, approval by the FDA would provide a basis for accepting botanicals into managed care formularies and for reimbursement by third-party payers. Practitioners integrating CAM into their practices worry about insurance coverage for similar reasons. They are concerned that CAM will become the "new" low-reimbursement insurance coverage therapy.

Q: What are the current barriers to managed care coverage of CAM?

A: As HMOs have added coverage for certain CAM, they have found that several issues must be addressed for adequate integration. Some of these concerns include

- Passive patients: the use of CAM requires active patient involvement. Some adults are comfortable with care being directed by their physician and are not prepared to take an active role in care decisions.
- Physician discomfort: some physicians are uncomfortable with CAM and the idea of the empowered patient. If they are planning to add CAM to medical practice, conventional providers must identify how they will prepare for a shift to CAM integration. For example, what additional knowledge, training, or guidance is necessary for the physician for integration to occur?
- Lack of physician referrals: many managed care plans still require physician referrals for treatment by other providers. If the primary provider disapproves of CAM, referrals may not occur.
- Financial issues: There is currently a lack of well-defined criteria for what insurance should or should not pay. Clear utilization management guidelines are not yet standard or widely available for CAM, which presents a challenge for HMOs to make appropriate care decisions.

Q: Is there health policy that supports the use of CAM?

A: Authoritative health policy or statements promoting particular CAM are based upon evidence-based findings from federal-level or international research. During the 1990s, the NIH published support of acupuncture for select health conditions. Soon after, many clinics began to offer acupuncture for those conditions. In recent years, studies were published that supported the use of the herbal therapy Echinacea for immune support to quickly relieve viral conditions. While no definitive health policy supports such use, it is not uncommon for a pediatric physician to recommend this supplement to parents of children suffering with frequent upper respiratory or ear problems. It is anticipated that as more research finds that various CAM are effective for specific health conditions, health policy will follow. In the meantime, during 2000, the White House established a commission to study and recommend how to address both healthcare practitioner and consumer education about CAM in the years ahead. During the last several years more research has focused on CAM and its use in chronic illness treatments.[2,3]

Q: Are any hospitals beginning to integrate CAM into their programs? Where?

A: In response to the remarkable growth in CAM by consumers, some hospitals and health systems in the United States are offering integrative medicine to their clients. The healthcare agencies sponsor special free-standing centers or services housed in a hospital or clinic wing that range from massage therapy to extensive complementary/integrative therapies. It is estimated that there were approximately 125 such hospital-sponsored programs in the United States by late 2001. **Table 2.2** lists the names and the size of several sponsored integrative centers that were surveyed as part of a benchmarking project in 2001.

Table 2.2   Hospital-Sponsored Integrative Centers from 2001 Benchmarking Survey

Sponsor	Size (square feet)
Mercy Health Partners (Cincinnati, OH)	14,000
NY Beth Israel (New York, NY)	13,000
Health Alliance (Cincinnati, OH)	11,000
Catholic Healthcare West (Phoenix, AZ)	10,000
Catholic Healthcare West (San Jose, CA)	3,600
Thomas Jefferson University Hospital (Philadelphia, PA)	2,600
Stanford Medical Center (Palo Alto, CA)	2,350
University of Massachusetts Memorial Healthcare (Worcester, MA)	2,600
George Washington University Medical Center (Washington, DC)	850

Source: Weeks J. Hospital-sponsored integrative clinics: an in-depth report. *Integr Med Consult.* 2001;3(10):R-1–R-8.

Healthcare system-sponsored integrative clinics are in their early years of development in the United States. It will be an exciting time ahead as holistic integration of care develops around the United States. As of late 2001, several specific types of modalities were offered at most integrative healthcare centers. These CAM modalities are listed in **Table 2.3**.

Table 2.3   Clinical Services or Integrative Practioner Type

Service	Percent (%)
Massage therapy	93
Group or health education	93
Acupuncture	89
Nutritional services	72
Yoga	70
Mind-body programs	70

(Continues)

Table 2.3   Clinical Services or Integrative Practioner Type (Continued)

Service	Percent (%)
Multi-week condition specific	67
Tai Chi	52
Natural pharmaceuticals	48
Homeopathy	37
Chiropractor	19
Naturopathic physician	15

Source: Weeks J. Hospital-sponsored integrative clinics: an in-depth report. *Integr Med Consult.* 2001;3(10):R-1–R-8.

Q: Does the FDA regulate supplements such as herbal therapy? Why not?

A: More than 500 herbal products are marketed in retail grocery and drug stores, mail order houses, and on the Internet, yet none of the products are regulated by the FDA. In 1994, Congress passed the Dietary Supplement Health and Education Act (DSHEA). The law grandfathered most herbal supplements into a new class of products labeled as "dietary supplements" which allowed them to remain on the market. In 2000, the FDA declared that statements that do not relate to disease may be placed on supplements.

Q: How does U.S. FDA regulation compare to other countries' regulation of supplements?

A: Germany has a long-standing Commission E, similar to the U.S. FDA, that regulates and oversees herbal therapy usage in that country. In Germany, many herbal products are used as "medications" and not considered fringe products. In France and England, if a plant has a history of use it is considered safe and effective, and in Canada, herbal therapies are reviewed for safety, but not for proven effectiveness. Prescriptions for herbal therapies are even covered by insurance in France, Germany, Italy, and Japan. Therefore, many medical practitioners in those countries routinely use alternative methods of healing, including herbal medications.

Q: Why don't some patients talk about their use of CAM with their medical providers?

A: One study found that up to 70% of people who use CAM therapies do not share this information with their healthcare provider, and many patients don't feel comfortable revealing their herbal supplement use to healthcare providers. Often questions are not asked because healthcare providers do not have adequate tools or methods to ask about CAM usage. Appropriate tools include assessment forms that include questions about CAM usage and use interview methods that elicit information in a nonjudgmental manner.

Q: What should healthcare providers ask about CAM use?

A: The healthcare provider should be prepared to discuss CAM choices with each patient, and assure that the patient is aware of known risks for a particular intervention. Current medical literature has suggested that practitioners of conventional therapies have an obligation to fully discuss the risks and benefits of CAM treatment, especially if the complementary treatment displaces conventional medical protocols. Consumers should not wait for a doctor to discuss these CAM therapy risks. It is important for all adults to take steps to learn about any therapy they are planning to use. Documentation of these discussions is essential.

Q: How does "informed consent" relate to CAM use?

A: All adults should be informed about any type of healthcare therapy practitioners plan to use, including safety issues, side effects, and other issues.[4-7] This includes CAM. Questions to consider before beginning any type of CAM therapy include

- What benefits can I expect from this therapy?
- What are the risks associated with this therapy?
- Do the benefits outweigh the risks for my disease or condition?
- What side effects can be expected?
- Will the therapy interfere with any of my daily activities?
- How long will I need to undergo treatment?
- How often will my progress or plan of treatment be assessed?
- Will I need to buy any equipment or supplies?
- Are there scientific articles or references about using the treatment for my condition?
- Could the therapy interact with conventional treatments?
- Are there any conditions for which this treatment should not be used?

To learn more about selecting a CAM practitioner, see the NCCAM's fact sheet, "Selecting a Complementary and Alternative Medicine Practitioner," available online at: **http://nccam.nih.gov/health/practitioner/index.htm**.

Q: Should patients tell healthcare practitioners if they use CAM? Why?

A: If you use any CAM therapy, inform your primary healthcare provider. This is for your safety and so your healthcare provider can develop a comprehensive treatment plan. Decisions about medical care and treatment should be made in consultation with a healthcare provider and based on the condition and needs of each person. Discuss information on CAM with your healthcare provider before making any decisions about treatment or care. An example of the seriousness of this can be seen with some herbs which act as anticoagulants and should be discontinued at least two weeks prior to surgery. Decisions about your healthcare are important, including decisions about whether to use CAM.

If you use any CAM therapy, inform your primary healthcare provider, and nurses who may work with you in clinical or acute areas. This is for your safety and so your healthcare provider can develop a comprehensive treatment plan.

If you take prescription medication and herbal therapies, discuss this with your pharmacy practitioner and your doctor. This is important to identify safety issues on using medicine and supplements.

Q: **What responsibility do nurses have in assessing the use of CAM?**

A: Many nurses realize that CAM are popular with many people and that certain therapies are often recommended for certain medical conditions, such as herbal supplements for osteoarthritis. Nurses have the responsibility and the skills necessary to assess a patient's patterns of CAM usage that may have an adverse affect on a patient's recovery from illness. Most state Boards of Nursing agree that the Registered Nurse is accountable to be a patient advocate in assessing a patient's use of CAM and educating patients about safety in CAM use. In a safe, supportive, empowering and nonjudgmental interaction, the nurse should ask open-ended questions such as "what things do you do to improve or maintain your health?"

Q: **What are the risk factors associated with use of CAM versus conventional medicine?**

A: Many experts suggest that in general, CAM therapies have less risk and side effects than conventional medicine. For example, many CAM therapies are external (massage, chiropractic, Tai Chi) unlike medical therapies that require ingestion of a drug, surgery, or infusion of intravenous medications.

The fact that a plant is natural does not automatically mean that the products made from that plant are innocuous and safe. Hundreds of herbal remedies are available today, many of which do not have well-documented research and publication of side effects and serious toxicity. In addition, patients with potentially life-threatening illness or serious symptoms are at risk when seeking herbal remedies while foregoing medical evaluation. In some instances, seeking medical advice earlier could mean the difference between life and death, as with atypical chest pains or bleeding.

Q: Are the elderly at any increased risk when using herbal supplements?

A: Yes, elderly individuals continue to face increased risk if using herbal supplements along with conventional drugs. Polypharmacy (the daily intake of multiple medications) is a problem for elders who consume more medications than any other age group. For example, although the elderly made up only 13% of the United States population as of late 1997, they used about 30% of all prescribed medications and 40% of all over the counter drugs.[8] As of late 2002, those figures remained constant, as reported by the University of North Carolina Program on Aging. This University hosts an informative website for consumers and practitioners concerned about the use of multiple medications, as listed in the Suggested Readings. Although the use of CAM is most prevalent in adults 25 to 49 (92% who report such use), nearly 40% of adults older than 50 report such use. All adults must remember that adverse reactions and interactions are much more likely when a person combines both prescription and herbal therapies.

Q: What types of CAM tend to be effective or selected for chronic health problems?

A: Many adults with chronic health conditions select various CAM for symptom management. The therapies commonly used for joint health and conditions such as arthritis are nutritional supplements such as chondroitin and glucosamine. People with generalized musculoskeletal conditions often claim to find relief through massage, chiropractic, acupuncture, or acupressure, as well as many other less common soft-tissue CAM therapies such as reflexology. While there are no CAM that "cure" chronic illness or provide conclusive symptom relief, there are multiple texts and websites that list CAM therapies suggested for various types of health condition. The National Center for Complementary and Alternative Medicine (NCCAM) also describes several studies for various diagnoses.

Futher information on NCCAM, as well as additional web sources for CAM, can be found in the Suggested Readings section of this chapter.

Suggested Readings

NCCAM Clearinghouse
    Toll-free: 1-888-644-6226
    International: 301-519-3153
    TTY (for deaf or hard-of-hearing callers): 1-866-464-3615
    E-mail: info@nccam.nih.gov
    Web site: http://nccam.nih.gov
    Address: NCCAM Clearinghouse, P.O. Box 7923, Gaithersburg, MD 20898-7923
    Fax: 1-866-464-3616
    Fax-on-Demand Service: 1-888-644-6226

Alternative Health News Online. Available at: http://www.altmedicine.com/

Herbs for Health. Available at: http://www.discoverherbs.com/

National Center for Complementary and Alternative Medicine. Available at:
    http://nccam.nih.gov/

University of North Carolina, School of Medicine, Program on Aging. How to avoid
    Polypharmacy, 2002. Available at: http://www.med.unc.edu/aging/polypharmacy/
    avoid.htm

References

1. Sarnat RL, Winterstein J. Clinical and cost outcomes of an integrative medicine IPA. *Journal of Manipulative & Physiological Therapeutics.* Jun 2004;27(5): 336–347.

2. Gordon JS. The White House Commission on Complementary and Alternative Medicine Policy and the future of healthcare. *Alternative Therapies in Health & Medicine.* Sep–Oct 2004;10(5):20–23.

3. McCarthy M. US panel calls for more support of alternative medicine. *Lancet.* Apr 6 2002;359(9313):1213.

4. Caspi O, Holexa J. Lack of standards in informed consent in complementary and alternative medicine. *Complementary Therapies in Medicine.* Jun 2005;13(2): 123–130.

5. Bulen JA, Jr. 2003 Greenwall Bioethics Award. Complementary and alternative medicine. Ethical and legal aspects of informed consent to treatment. *Journal of Legal Medicine.* Sep 2003;24(3):331–358.

6. Sugarman J. Informed consent, shared decision-making, and complementary and alternative medicine. *Journal of Law, Medicine & Ethics.* 2003;31(2):247–250.

7. Monaco GP, Smith G. Informed consent in complementary and alternative medicine: current status and future needs. *Seminars in Oncology.* Dec 2002;29(6):601–608.

8. University of North Carolina, School of Medicine, Program on Aging. Available at: www.med.unc.edu/wrkunits/3ctrpgm/aging/welcome. Accessed October 25, 2005.

3

Ethics and Complementary and Alternative Medicine

Mary Cipriano Silva, RN, FAAN

James J. Fletcher, PhD

About the Authors

Mary Cipriano Silva is a clinical professor in the School of Public Health and Health Sciences at the University of Massachusetts Amherst. She is a prolific writer in the area of bioethics and was a member of the American Nurses Association task force that wrote the current *Code of Ethics for Nurses with Interpretive Statements*. Her research focuses on the ethics of managed care.

James J. Fletcher is a professor emeritus of philosophy in the Department of Philosophy at George Mason University where he specializes in bioethics and is the ethics collaborator in the Office of Health Care Ethics in the College of Nursing and Health Sciences. In addition to research and teaching in bioethics, he is a member of the Ethics Committee and chair of the Human Research Review Committee for a community hospital. He sits on the institutional review board for a biotechnology company and serves as a member of data and safety monitoring boards for the National Institutes of Health.

Q: What got you interested in CAM and ethics?

A: At 16, Silva's father, now 98, became a devotee of a holistic healthy life style that involved CAM. To this day, he uses positive thinking, dietary supplements, and chiropractors. However, for most of his life, CAM had been "put down" by conventional healthcare practitioners because they were outside of allopathic practices. Being closed minded about CAM, however, has ethical implications because harm by omission can occur. We believe that omitting CAM when it could clearly benefit, and not harm, patients is wrong.

Q: How do the ethics of conventional practitioners and CAM practitioners vary?

A: Underlying ethical philosophies vary. If we were conventional practitioners, we would be committed to not harming patients, respecting them, and being fair to them. We also would be committed to patients' rights and our duties to ensure these rights. If we were CAM practitioners, we would be committed to helping patients attain inner wholeness and a connection with the universe that involves their mind, body, and spirit. We also would be committed to the ethics inherent in spirituality, caring, and healing. Both conventional practitioners and CAM practitioners ascribe to doing good, preventing harm, and removing harm.[1]

Q: How do codes of ethics relate to CAM?

A: Codes of ethics express a profession's highest standards as determined not only by the profession's values, but also by what a profession owes members of a society. Regarding CAM, we, as healthcare providers, value and owe society freedom from harm, honesty, caring, healing when possible, integrity, and advocacy, to name a few. We, as healthcare providers, also value and owe society a commitment that we will not bow to pressure from other persons, institutions, or laws to do harm regarding CAM.

Q: What codes of ethics relate to CAM?

A: We believe that all healthcare codes of ethics, either explicitly or implicitly, relate to CAM. Some ethics codes from a variety of organizations have identified important ethical concepts:
- *American Holistic Medical Association (AHMA) Principles of Ethics:* treating the total person: body, mind, and spirit; improving skills and medical knowledge; determining the effectiveness and safety of all methods of treatment; acquiring the skills and training necessary for the delivery of care.
- *American Chiropractic Association (ACA) Code of Ethics:* showing loyalty, compassion, and respect for patients; ensuring that clinical judgments and practices are objective and solely for the patient's benefit; promoting health, preventing illness, and alleviating suffering.

- *International Council of Nurses (ICN) Code of Ethics for Nurses:* promoting health; alleviating suffering; gaining spiritual awareness; giving nonprejudicial nursing care; accepting social responsibility; taking care of the natural environment.
- *American Nurses Association (ANA) Code of Ethics for Nurses with Interpretive Statements:* providing universal and nonprejudicial nursing care; alleviating suffering; understanding that patients come first; preserving nurses' unity of character; accepting social responsibility; taking care of the work and natural environment.
- *American Holistic Nurses' Association (AHNA) Position Statement on Holistic Nursing Ethics:* all of the preceding, plus accepting mind-body-spirit unity; healing; nurturing co-workers; applying holistic nursing theories; maintaining the ecosystem.

Q: What standards of practice related to CAM are used?

A: We use the *American Holistic Nurses' Association Standards of Holistic Nursing Practice.*[2] These standards include core values such as holistic ethics, holistic self-care, and holistic caring. Keep in mind that standards of practice relate to ethics because they identify right conduct.

Q: What ethical theories relate to CAM?

A: Three ethical theories are relevant to CAM and are used to interpret and judge human actions in terms of right and wrong.

Utilitarian ethical theory judges actions strictly in terms of the consequences of our actions. Those actions that produce the greatest amount of happiness are right; those actions that tend to increase the amount of unhappiness are wrong. Obviously, health tends to increase happiness and illness decreases it. Therefore, the success of promoting and using CAM can certainly be judged by the utilitarian standard. For example, it would be wrong to continue to advertise a dietary supplement that failed to contribute to health or general well being.

Virtue ethical theory focuses on the character of individuals rather than on the moral quality of individual actions. Those individuals who develop certain traits, called virtues, can be expected to act in ways that fulfill us as human beings. Thus, virtue ethics would stress traits such as being honest, compassionate, and just in one's dealings with others regarding CAM.

Care ethical theory focuses on the moral responsibility for relationships related to caring and to our pursuit of happiness. Many alternative therapies (e.g., therapeutic touch) may be disregarded or underappreciated if one fails to follow the care theory requirement to recognize and respect the importance of relationships.

Q: What ethical principles relate to CAM?

A: The dominant principles of contemporary bioethics are nonmaleficence, beneficence, distributive justice, and autonomy. All of these apply to CAM.

Nonmaleficence is our obligation to "do no wrong." For example, you should not make recommendations that exceed your knowledge or make claims that are clearly exaggerated or not substantiated. More importantly, you have an obligation to warn clients about possible adverse interactions between alternative substances and prescribed medications. Since many of these substances are not studied or approved by the Food and Drug Administration (FDA), practitioners have a particular obligation to learn what they can about possible interactions.

Beneficence requires that one acts on behalf of the interests of others. Professional healthcare workers have a clear obligation of beneficence towards their patients. If, for example, CAM seems to be effective for certain chronic conditions, beneficence obliges you to make this information available to your clients. When dealing with members of diverse cultures, you have an obligation to learn what they may be using in the way of alternative therapies and to monitor their interaction with biomedical therapies.

Most CAM is paid out of pocket. This means that many useful therapies may be out of reach of those on limited budgets. This raises questions of distributive justice that our society has an obligation to address.

Finally, by the principle of autonomy, individuals should freely choose a plan to meet their health needs. Of central importance in making a free choice is the information one requires to make an informed choice. So, autonomy requires that individuals who advocate CAM supply complete information about the product, including what it is likely to accomplish and how it will affect those who take it.

Q: How does ethics relate to dietary supplements?

A: We believe that ethics relate to dietary supplements when safety is an issue. As previously noted, many dietary supplements (e.g., vitamins) are not carefully regulated by the FDA. Consequently, manufacturers of dietary supplements too often use misleading advertising to promise more benefits than the supplement can deliver. In addition, many manufacturers add substances to dietary supplements that have no nutritional value but drive up the cost of the supplements. Finally, manufacturers do not always identify the side effects or drug interactions that may occur with use of dietary supplements or, if identified, they are found in the fine print and are difficult to read. All of the preceding tactics may harm patients.[3]

Q: How does ethics relate to spirituality?

A: Until recent years, ethics and spirituality were often viewed differently. We believe that commonalities exist, for example, both ethics and spirituality are grounded in values. Ethics seeks to clarify desirable values that deal with the right or the good in life; spirituality seeks to clarify desirable values that deal with the sacred or the Absolute in life. That which focuses on the right or the good in life often also focuses on the sacred or the Absolute in life.

Q: How does ethics relate to spiritual practices?

A: Perhaps the most common ethical and spiritual principle deals with how we treat others, especially those persons whose values, socioeconomic status, or cultures are different from our own. How we treat others leads to the principle of respect for persons, whereby all persons, regardless of defining attributes, are viewed as unconditionally worthy human beings. The principle of respect for persons includes ethical and spiritual practices such as

- helping persons to find meaning in life;
- giving hope;
- demonstrating caring;
- giving due consideration to perspectives different from one's own;
- appreciating other persons; and
- connecting with other persons, animals, and/or the environment.

    In addition, spiritual assessment tools have become more common in practice. We personally do not like these tools because they typically are developed by healthcare providers from their restrictive perspective. Instead, we prefer obtaining life narratives that include ethics and spirituality from the perspectives of the patient's life.

Q: How does ethics relate to prayer and healing?

A: We, along with many healthcare providers involved in CAM, believe that prayer can positively affect healing and, thus, is an ethical good. In addition, considerable empirical research supports the hypothesis that prayer promotes at least some positive health outcomes. Nevertheless, the following points represent some ethical considerations:

- that there should not be an incongruity of type of healing desired between the pray-er(s) and the one(s) prayed for;
- that the pray-er(s) never pray for bad or evil outcomes for the one(s) prayed for; and
- that false hope through deceptive prayer practices about healing is never given to the one(s) prayed for.

Prayer to promote healing in nursing was first grounded in the writings of Florence Nightingale. Not until recently have the interconnections among prayer, healing, health, and ethics been given the considerations they deserve (see Chapter 14).

Q: How does ethics relate to nontraditional practitioners?

A: Many nontraditional practitioners are not included in traditional professional codes of ethics, for example, those of the American Medical Association or the American Nurses Association. Nonetheless, a CAM practitioner is still subject to standards of ethics. In some cases there are practitioner standards such as those for chiropractors, but even in the absence of a related association that formulates standards, individuals who directly sell a product or contract to provide a service are subject to societal standards for business. In particular, one is required to be honest in advertising a product or service, to have sufficient knowledge and competent skills in providing the service, and to provide sufficient information so that a potential client may make an informed decision.

Q: How does informed consent relate to CAM and research ethics?

A: If we were to conduct a research study related to CAM, one of our first steps would be to obtain an informed consent from study participants. The primary reasons for this step are to determine capacity for consent and to disclose all information considered material to the informed consent decision. Capacity for consent is important because it tells us whether or not a prospective study participant comprehends what is being disclosed. If the prospective study participant clearly does not comprehend what is being disclosed, it would be unethical of us to include the person in a CAM study unless we obtained a proxy consent. Overall, healthcare providers do a good job of disclosing pertinent information related to a research study but do a poor job of assessing comprehension of that information. Without comprehension, the potential for harm and the violation of a person's wholeness occurs.[4,5]

Q: How does selection of research participants relate to CAM and research ethics?

A: In CAM studies, researchers must determine the number of participants needed and their defining characteristics. The number of participants needed could be so large that scarce resources (e.g., the researchers, the monies available) are depleted, thus, the ethics of fairness are compromised. The number of participants available could be so small that the validity of the study is questioned and important information about CAM could not be implemented into practice. Regarding defining characteristics of the research participants, ethical issues could occur by omission or commission. We could omit from our CAM study persons who should be included but are not (e.g., persons of only one gender when the CAM being studied involves both genders) or, we could include in our CAM study persons who should not be included (e.g., vulnerable participants who would not benefit from the CAM study).

Q: How do research designs relate to CAM and research ethics?

A: The two major categories of research designs are quantitative research designs and qualitative research designs, each of which presents ethical challenges in CAM research. In quantitative CAM research, especially experimental designs, researchers should rarely use an experimental CAM treatment that could cause more than minimal harm to study participants. Also, if researchers offer a known beneficial CAM treatment to experimental participants, but not to control participants, they would be in violation of research ethics. In qualitative CAM research, because of the sensitive and in-depth nature of many of the topics explored, researchers must be exceedingly conscientious in preserving research participants' anonymity. Also, with in-depth qualitative designs, focusing on the researchers' life narratives rather than the study participants' life narratives violates the ethical principle of respect for persons. In both quantitative and qualitative CAM research, researchers must avoid scientific misconduct, including such ethical violations as plagiarism, data fabrication, data falsification, and data manipulation to obtain desired results.[6]

Q: How does dissemination of research results relate to CAM and research ethics?

A: If we have conducted a rigorous study related to CAM, we should present or publish the results to benefit our patients and our profession. If we are coauthoring a manuscript about our CAM study, we should give proper credit to coauthors in accord with their contributions to the manuscript. We also should ensure that all persons who contributed to the study understand the ethical ramifications of plagiarism. If you paraphrase other persons' words, directly use their words, or use their organizational format, you must give them credit. If you do not do so, you have committed plagiarism, and plagiarism could destroy your reputation and your career. Never, never, be tempted!

Q: How does culture affect ethical values in CAM?

A: One's culture fashions a worldview, so what you appreciate or value is, in large measure, a product of your culture. In a homogenous society there is wide agreement about the practices and products to be valued. The United States is a pluralistic society and there is a wide range of cultural beliefs and values shared by members of our society. One value is health, but health may be understood in different ways depending on one's cultural perspective.

The dominant Western perspective of health is based on the biomedical model. It relies on science and prefers a systemic approach to healing. Other cultures hold a more holistic or integrative perspective, seeing a person's health as involving mind, body, and spirit. The holistic perspective gives rise to many of the therapies included under CAM. The struggle to recognize the value of CAM, in large measure, is a clash of cultures. Only when the scientific culture opens itself to other methods of healing will the values of these alternative therapies be adequately assessed.

Q: How do culture and ethics relate to CAM?

A: Within the American culture, the two ethical principles most related to culture and CAM are respect for persons and nonmaleficence (do no harm). Because our culture is so diverse, misunderstandings about various types of health practices related to CAM can easily occur. If mainstream American healthcare providers believe that they know which CAM is best for persons of other cultures without talking with them, they not only are guilty of ethnocentrism but also of violation of the ethical principle of respect for persons. On the other hand, if these providers accept and implement without question the CAM of another culture, they could harm patients. Therefore, taking into consideration such factors as legitimate biological differences, family and social norms, and patterns of communication, you must decide where to draw the line between respect for persons and not harming them. For example, you might allow certain prayer rituals (respect for persons), but not allow the use of herbs that interact negatively with a patient's diet or drug regimen (not harming persons).

Q: What do you do when ethical values regarding CAM conflict?

A: Society is based on the assumption of human dignity. Fundamentally, you recognize the dignity of others when you respect their right to think and act for themselves. As noted, cultural differences can lead to a wide variety of beliefs and practices regarding health care. Professional healthcare workers have an obligation to respect the cultural differences that their patients represent. Dismissing their practices without learning why they have undertaken them is disrespectful and fails to honor their human dignity. A healthcare professional may believe not only that a practice is not helpful, but also even dangerous to the patient, unless supplemented with other techniques. Respecting diversity does not mean that one should abandon professional standards. It does require that you listen to your patient with an open mind. It also requires that you see the importance of the alternative measure as a cultural response and not just a physical response to the illness you are treating.

Q: Who should have access to CAM?

A: Part of respecting human dignity is acknowledging autonomy. Any competent adult should have access to CAM as part of his or her health regimen. If a person does not have sufficient money to purchase CAM, ethical and creative means should be sought so that distributive justice is ensured.

Q: Who should pay for CAM?

A: Currently, most expenditures for CAM are out of pocket. Some services, like acupuncture or chiropractic adjustments, are covered to some extent by insurance. Other services like aromatherapy or guided imagery are not usually covered. Many diet supplements are sold over the counter and are an out-of-pocket expense. The issue of healthcare costs in the United States has not been dealt with adequately at the legislative or societal level. Until we as a society decide what a minimum standard for health coverage should be and how we will address the needs of the millions of citizens who lack any form of health coverage, the question of who should pay for CAM will probably not be addressed. Whenever it is addressed, some basic issues will have to be considered. For example, what type of evidence will be required to demonstrate that the substance or procedure accomplishes its objectives? Who will have oversight and control over the claims made on behalf of herbal substances? These are not impossible hurdles; in Europe and Asia, for example, herbal and other complementary therapies have been integrated with biomedicine for some time.

Q: What are some ethical decision-making frameworks that you can apply to the ethics of CAM?

A: In a general sense, all ethical decision-making frameworks can be applied to the ethics of CAM because they follow the steps of a basic problem-solving process. This process includes

- Collect data relevant to patient context (e.g., diagnosis, social norms, cultural background) and CAM;
- Analyze ethical issues within patient context, relevant collected data, ethical knowledge base, and CAM;
- Plan viable options within patient context, relevant collected data, ethical knowledge base, and CAM;
- Select viable options to implement based on patient context, relevant collected data, ethical knowledge base, and CAM; and
- Evaluate the degree to which viable options resolved or failed to resolve ethical issues related to CAM.

In the preceding ethical decision-making framework, *ethical knowledge base* refers to, but is not limited to, the ethical theories and principles discussed above. Note that in practice, the steps of the ethical decision-making framework are often not linear. For example, after you have analyzed the ethical issues, you may need to collect more data, or, after you have evaluated the degree to which the viable options were attained, or not attained, you may need to select another plan of action.

Q: Should healthcare providers ever compromise their own conscience when dealing with CAM?

A: Overall, we believe that healthcare providers should not compromise their conscience when dealing with CAM or with any other healthcare practices and procedures. A compromised conscience can lead to moral distress, which often manifests itself as painful psychological (e.g., guilt) or physiological (e.g., insomnia) signs or symptoms. Before you take an implacable stand on ethical issues, including those related to CAM, you should consider the following questions:

- How did I get myself into a position where I felt pressured to compromise my conscience?
- Have I listened with a truly open mind to those persons who believe differently than I do?
- Can I find common ground between how I believe and how other healthcare providers believe regarding the same ethical issue?
- Could my implacable stand, as opposed to principled compromise, cause more harm than good to those persons I serve?
- Could my implacable stand result in abandonment of a patient?

After considering questions such as the preceding ones, you should be in a better position to cope with issues of conscience.

Q: How can healthcare providers be better prepared to handle ethical issues when working with CAM?

A: The preceding text of this chapter should give you some ideas on how you can be better prepared to handle ethical issues related to CAM. Some of our other thoughts are:

- Conduct an assessment of your own values, including acknowledgment of those areas where you may feel intolerant toward others.
- Prepare yourself with a background in healthcare ethics, especially ethical theories and principles, scope and standards of practice, and codes of ethics.
- Attend conferences and seminars on ethics and CAM.
- Discuss ethical concerns related to CAM with healthcare colleagues.
- Keep abreast of the latest thinking in health care and CAM via credible web sites (e.g., the National Institutes of Health's site on CAM. Available at: http://nccam.nih.gov/).

Q: Where can you learn more about ethics and CAM?

A: One article that discusses both ethics and CAM is Silva and Ludwick's "Ethical issues in complementary alternative therapies."

Three good books on understanding ethical theories, principles, and/or approaches to ethical decision making are *Principles of Biomedical Ethics*, *The Basics of Bioethics*, and *A Practical Companion to Ethics*.

Form more information on the books and the journal article mentioned above, as well as the ANA Center for Ethics and Human Rights, see this chapter's Suggested Readings section (p. 32).

Suggested Readings

JOURNALS

Silva MC, Ludwick R. Ethical issues in complementary/alternative therapies. November 1, 2001. *Online Journal of Issues in Nursing.* Available at: http://www.nursingworld.org/ojin/ethics_7.htm. Accessed June 16, 2005.

BOOKS

Beauchamp TL, Childress JF. *Principles of Biomedical Ethics.* 5th ed. New York, NY: Oxford University Press; 2001.

Veatch RM. *The Basics of Bioethics.* 2nd ed.. Upper Saddle River, NJ: Prentice Hall; 2003.

Weston A. *A Practical Companion to Ethics.* 2nd ed. New York, NY: Oxford University Press; 2002.

ANA CODE OF ETHICS FOR NURSES

American Nurses Association. *Code of Ethics for Nurses with Interpretive Statements.* Washington, DC: American Nurses Publishing; 2001.

  800-274-4ANA (4262)

The Center for Ethics and Human Rights. Available at: www.ana.org/ethics/.

References

1. Lim B, Schmidt K, White A, Ernst E. Reporting of ethical standards: differences between complementary and orthodox medicine journals? *Wiener Klinische Wochenschrift.* Jul 31 2004;116(14):500–503.

2. Frisch N, Dossey B, Guzetta C, Quinn J. *The Standard of Holsitic Nursing Practice and How They're Applied in Daily Practice.* New York: Jones and Bartlett; 2000.

3. Egan CD. Addressing use of herbal medicine in the primary care setting. *Journal of the American Academy of Nurse Practitioners.* Apr 2002;14(4):166–171.

4. Brophy E. Does a doctor have a duty to provide information and advice about complementary and alternative medicine? *Journal of Law & Medicine.* Feb 2003; 10(3):271–284.

5. Weir M. Obligation to advise of options for treatment—medical doctors and complementary and alternative medicine practitioners. *Journal of Law & Medicine.* Feb 2003;10(3):296–307.

6. Gorman RF. Obstacles to research in complementary and alternative medicine. *Medical Journal of Australia.* Jan 19 2004;180(2):95; author reply 95–96.

4

The Influence of Culture in Complementary and Alternative Medicine

Lyn Freeman, PhD

About the Author

Lyn Freeman is a specialist in the research, education, and integration of Complementary and Alternative Medicine in educational and healthcare settings. She is chair of Integrative Health Studies for Saybrook Graduate School in San Francisco and president of Mind Matters Research, an Alaskan organization dedicated to research with Imagery as treatment for chronic disease. Dr. Freeman is currently performing research that assesses the effects of imagery practice, Buddhist chanting, and Alaskan traditional healer treatments on the human biofield. She is also conducting a study for the National Cancer Institute to evaluate the effects of imagery on recovering breast cancer patients.

Q: How did you become interested in CAM?

A: Over the course of my life, I have been exposed to many cultures and witnessed a variety of healing and spiritual practices. As long as I can remember, I have been fascinated by the role that culture, ritual, and ceremony play in molding the mind, healing the body, and nurturing the spirit.

During the first half of life, my experience with alternative medicine was mostly related to cultural mind-body practices. I was most interested in meditation practices related to mystical states of consciousness. Later, I was interested in how imagery was used culturally for alleviation of disease and for invoking altered states of consciousness.

Q: How did culture begin to play a role in your practice?

A: I began to study the Coptic mystical tradition, Alaskan Native traditional healing, Surat Shabd Yoga, shamanic traditions, and Buddhism. I was fascinated by the fact that certain priests, gurus, masters, and teachers were able to control their bodies because they had learned to control their minds. In some cultures, practitioners learned mindfulness through meditation. They learned the power of internal imagery. They learned how to control the biofields around their body and the body of their patients. All of this played a part in crafting what I do in my practice today.

I first studied the teachings of the Coptic Philosophy and later met the Egyptian seven-ring Coptic master, Hamid Bey. Hamid Bey taught me that anyone can master their minds and bodies but few ever put in the effort to do so. I had some amazing healing experiences during very difficult life transition points. I would say those experiences were the beginning of my realization of how powerful mind-body effects could be for those who are willing to put in the effort and commitment.

Q: How does culture play a role in the use of CAM and health care?

A: Every culture has its own beliefs on how or what cures and heals. While it is not possible to understand the teachings of every culture, it is important as healthcare providers that we respect the cultural teachings of our patients when they enter into the healthcare arena. Whether we see our patients in birthing rooms, long-term care facilities, acute care settings, or the home environment, culture will play a profound part in how well they heal. In this country, with rare exception, the patient will choose how they want to be treated medically. Inquiring into and showing respect for a patient's culture will assist the healthcare professional in treating the patient most effectively.

Q: Where did your experiences lead you in studying different cultural traditions and CAM?

A: At mid-life, I went back to school and earned advanced degrees in human sciences and psychology. The masters in human sciences degree allowed me to explore in more depth a variety of the cultural traditions that had always interested me: shamanic healing, traditional healing, Ayurvedic medicine and psychology, and Buddhist meditation techniques to name a few. I was privileged to study with Ruth-Inge Heinze, a well-known researcher and shaman in two cultures and Stanley Krippner, a leading expert on shamanic traditions and altered states of consciousness. Stanley became my mentor and friend. The work he has done throughout his life has inspired much of what I do today.

While earning the Ph.D. in psychology, I studied psychoneuro-immunology and mind-body interventions—relaxation, meditation, hypnosis, and imagery specifically—as they related to the treatment of chronic disease. I performed research with chronic patients suffering from asthma. We utilized imagery to reduce their symptoms and modulate immune and physiological responses, specifically the inflammatory and broncho-restrictive aspects of asthma. Subjects significantly improved their symptoms, as compared to a control group and a wait-list group. Much of the imagery that can improve or worsen conditions like asthma is engrained in our cultural attitudes and even our cultural myths. As I work with traditional healers today, I see healing imagery woven into every aspect of what they do. Their imagery is, of course, culturally based.

Q: When we talk about culture, what do we really mean and how can that influence healthcare practices?

A: Culture is not only about race and ethnicity. Culture influences how we relate to age, gender, sexuality, and disabilities among other things. For example, Alaska native traditions have great respect for their elders and for the wisdom that age and experience bring. As long as elders are able to remain in their villages, surrounded by the love and respect of their families, they can maintain productive lives for many years. When they are removed for "medical reasons" from the village and placed in long-term care facilities, their lives are cut short. They will, quite literally, turn their faces to the wall and die. I have seen this happen.

Much of the evolving culture in the United States worships youth and sexuality. Relatively young people will undertake life threatening surgery to look younger. On the other hand, they may refuse life saving surgery because it would cause some level of disfigurement. One is a traditional culture; the other an evolving culture. Culture still affects how we make medical decisions, how we heal, and how we choose to die.

Q: Do you believe that CAM really works?

A: This is a very broad question. When practiced by healers who are well-steeped in the history, philosophy, mechanisms, and methods of a particular discipline, and when these forms of intervention are then offered to the appropriate body of patients, yes they certainly do work. I will admit a bias here. I like to see CAM that comes from the cultural traditions offered by persons fully trained in those traditions. For example, I favor the type of acupuncture offered by a Traditional Chinese Medicine (TCM) practitioner. The French version of acupuncture taught to licensed physicians is more limited in scope and physicians will typically lack the lifetime of continuing hands-on experience that you find in a full-time TCM practitioner. Just as conventional medicine is both a science and an art, so is the delivery of CAM. You must know your treatment in great depth and have practiced it for many years to become highly effective.

I prefer to see dietary and herbal preparations provided by those trained and licensed in TCM or the Ayurvedic forms of medicine, since these cultural healing traditions consider all aspects of the persons' health and treat the whole person. I like to see meditation practices taught by those involved in the full philosophy underlying that practice. Buddhist Mindfulness Meditation should be taught by those who live what they teach. The same applies to Transcendental Meditation (TM). This form of meditation is the most researched method in the world today and it produces incredibly good outcomes. Part of this is no doubt because only those persons who live the TM lifestyle and meditate and teach on a continuous basis are certified to be instructors.

Q: Is there research to support CAM?

A: In the past two decades, I have personally reviewed more than 10,000 clinical applications of various CAM: relaxation, meditation, hypnosis, imagery, biofeedback, acupuncture, chiropractic, homeopathy, massage, herbal medicine, and spiritual healing practices. When studies are well designed, when they reflect the original practices, are delivered correctly by trained and experienced practitioners, and when they are provided to the right patient population, you bet they work. Take out any of the above components— a badly designed study, a poorly trained practitioner, use of a method that is contradictory to the original healing tradition—and the outcomes will demonstrate no efficacy at all and may even cause harm. One of the problems with many of our early research studies was that the researchers worked very hard on designing a good study by Western model standards, but then performed a study that didn't reflect the traditional treatment at all, nor were the treatments necessarily delivered to the population that historically had been demonstrated to benefit from that form of CAM.

Q: **What are the biggest differences you see by cultures in the use of CAM?**

A: I would first like to address what the different cultures seem to have in common. The "original" forms of healing (Ayurvedic, Chinese, Alaska Native and American Indian Traditional healing, Shamanism, to name a few) all emphasized the treatment of the whole person (mind, body, and spirit), and even further, of the community. The community and family were always part of the healing process. The use of herbal medications, manipulations (forms of massage and spinal adjustment), and dietary practices were part of the healing practice. Spiritual practices were also fundamental. It might be energy healing, meditation, prayer, imagery, story-telling, ceremony, ritual, or cleansing practices that were unique to that culture, but the spiritual practices of healing were always there.

Cultures differ in relation to CAM depending on where the culture resides. Some herbal treatments might be more popular than others. This is dependent on what is naturally available. Our traditional healers in Alaska become highly irritated when outsiders think all traditional healers should be alike. They remind outsiders that their practices evolve just as other disciplines do.

Q: **How does traditional healing delivered by Indigenous persons fit into CAM?**

A: I have had the privilege of knowing, observing, and becoming friends with many Alaska Native traditional healers. Like other cultures, they have their own "specializations" and different traditional healers have different gifts. In Anchorage, the most respected healer in the state is a master of herbology and energy healing. She knows how to "turn babies," manipulate and massage, and how to heal soul wounds. She might be considered a generalist, in that she embodies all the traits typically found in traditional healers across the state. In Kotzebue, the healers are specialists in spinal manipulation and massage; they also use herbal treatments and practice minor forms of surgery. They work with a technique called poking and may lance wounds. Some also apply pressure to energy points, something like acupressure.

Traditional healing differs from some other healing systems in that you must be "called" to be a healer. It is not a situation where you can just receive education in how to be a traditional healer. You may be born with a gift, you may undergo a life transitioning experience (e.g., near-death) that prepares you to be a healer, and you will most often apprentice with another recognized healer. True traditional healers in Alaska are recognized by the elders to be healers. In Alaska, several of the tribal governments have incorporated traditional healers into their conventional medical care systems. There are traditional healer programs in Anchorage, Kotzebue, on the Kenai Peninsula, and in other parts of the state. Traditional healers who practice there are given the title of tribal doctor. However, being designated a tribal doctor does not mean you are always an accepted traditional healer. Community elders must recognize and validate the healer. Among the indigenous peoples in other states, some of the same "rules" apply. You must be called or chosen to heal, and it is the elders who will know who a true healer is.

Q: How do folk medicine, faith healing, and herbs play a role in culture and CAM?

A: These were all our original forms of medicine. Folk medicines were the forms of healing used before conventional medicine practices. Folk medicine was often practiced by wise women. In some countries, those healers were called witches and killed for their healing practices. Faith healing can be a powerful form of medicine. We now know from the research in psychoneuroimmunology and the studies of religious practices that faith can quite literally alter your immune and physiological responses. If we could bottle faith and give it in doses when needed much of the rest of our medicines would be unnecessary. We can't do that so easily, however. Herbal medicines have always been a mainstay of cultural healing practices. They were our first medicines, and many of our current-day pharmaceuticals evolved from the study of plants and their constituents.

Q: Does spirituality and spiritual beliefs play a role in culture and CAM?

A: Definitely. Just look at the explosion of research in the medical community related to spiritual healing practices. As our Western society became highly scientific and technically oriented, it lost much of its spiritual roots. Research by d'Quili and Newberg[1] has demonstrated that we are "hard wired" for spiritual experiences. In other words, we need a spiritual belief system and spiritual practices to be healthy and whole as human beings. We will seek out spiritual experiences one way or another. Culture, and the spiritual expressions embedded in each cultural system, provides us with a framework for religious and spiritual expression. Today, these belief systems overlap between cultures. The United States was founded on the principles of freedom of religion, but that religious freedom was originally framed within Christian traditions.

Today, we all have faiths within our culture: Judaism, Buddhism, Islam, and Hinduism to name a few. In our current world, acceptance of each other's spiritual freedom and quest for spirituality leads to peaceful coexistence, and a clash of cultural of spiritual expression leads to terrorism and war. In many ways, CAM helps us to come together in relationship to cultural differences. Learning how other cultures view healing also reveals how they express their spiritual side. Understanding leads to acceptance of diversity and acceptance of individual differences. Acceptance of individual differences can lead to healing and to peace.

Q: How do we merge the use of CAM, culture, and the science of allopathic medicine?

A: We begin by understanding the cultural roots of the different practices. There are many ways that individuals are attempting to merge CAM with allopathic medicine. The term "integrative medicine" has been employed to suggest that they are merging, but in many cases, this term has come to mean allopathic physicians utilizing some small, but fractured part of a cultural practice in their own medical practice. For example, the French form of acupuncture is employed by many physicians after receiving several hundred hours of training. This is only one small part of a true healing system. Many TCM practitioners are horrified by this approach. A cultural healing system is meant to treat the whole person and no "piece" should be isolated from the rest of the healing components of that system. In Western medicine, the approach is to deal with "pieces": organs, symptoms, surgical procedures. I am strongly opposed to this reductionist approach as a way for integrating cultural methods of healing. I am, however, a strong supporter of the "teaming" approach. For example, a patient may be triaged by an MD, a TCM practitioner, a nutritionist, an exercise physiologist, and a mind-body specialist who is a practitioner of a particular form of meditation or yoga practice. In this way, the body, mind, and spirit are considered. If finances do not allow for this type of intervention, then the programs should "stand alone" so that they maintain their integrity. The patient can then choose the forms of help that is appropriate. Utilization studies of CAM clearly demonstrate that patients do not pick CAM over conventional care. Rather, they utilize conventional care alongside other forms of treatment. Since there is the potential for adverse reactions between these systems, conventional and unconventional practitioners alike must ask their patients what types of treatments and products they are using and prescribe accordingly. In our country and in other countries, a new medical "culture" is evolving, where conventional medicine and unconventional medicine systems must come to terms with each other. Consumers will not allow one to win out over the other; they insist on having access to both forms of healing.

Q: How do I learn all the cultural beliefs and ethnic practices I need to know to make sure I do not offend a patient or separate them from their own cultural practices?

A: I don't think anyone can learn all the practices that exist. You avoid offending patients by being respectful of them and their family members. Remember to be respectful, not condescending of elders in each society. Then you ask your patient about what cultural practices they might be using, and you demonstrate by your attitude and your concern that you will not look down upon, nor be critical of, their cultural ways of healing. If you succeed in doing this, you will be able to work with patients of all cultures without offending them. It is also important to remember that in many cultures, family members speak for an ill elder or child. Do not dismiss the input of family members who can be very helpful in this regard.

Q: What type of research has been done in relation to culture and CAM?

A: There is more research than you might think. The research that is most culturally "pure" consists of the anecdotal reports, case studies, and observational studies. However, the experimental research on other forms of healing has exploded in the last decade. I would suggest reading *Mosby's Complementary and Alternative Medicine*[2] that surveys the research in 18 different categories. The history and philosophy sections in each chapter point the reader to the cultures that practice those forms of healing.

Q: Is there anything else you can recommend about this information?

A: There are research journals dedicated to individual forms of healing. I suggest searching pubmed.com and other research sites by topic. The National Center for Complementary and Alternative Medicine website (http://nccam.nih.gov), part of National Institute of Health, is the best place to see what research is currently underway or recently completed. That website also provides the reader with information on how to contact the different cultural centers related to research. Another good website for the review of herbal remedies is www.naturaldatabase.com, but you must pay a fee to be a member of this website. It is updated daily based on new findings in herbal and biomolecular research.

References

1. d'Aquili E, Newberg A. *The Mystical Mind: Probing the Biology of Religious Experience.* Minneapolis, MN: Fortress Press; 1999.

2. Freeman LW. *Mosby's Complementary and Alternative Medicine: A Research-Based Approach.* 2nd ed. St. Louis, MO: Mosby; 2004.

5

Education Clinical Issues in Complementary and Alternative Medicine

H. Lea Barbato Gaydos, PhD, RN, CNS, AHN-BC

About the Author

H. Lea Barbato Gaydos teaches at the University of Colorado, Colorado Springs, Beth-El College of Nursing and Health Sciences. Her areas of expertise include psychiatric/mental health nursing, holistic nursing, community health nursing, and aesthetics and the creative process. She is also a professional visual artist and has had many group exhibitions and three solo exhibitions. Dr. Gaydos' study and research interests focus on the life stories of healers, particularly nurses, and healing as experienced through creativity, spirituality, and aesthetics. In her practice she works with people to co-create their life stories in a Life Journey Portrait and with organizations to facilitate organizational change through aesthetic and creative processes.

Q: What got you interested in CAM?

A: At first glance this seems like a straight-forward question. Surely, there is a single thing I can point to or a discrete moment in time I can say was the beginning of my interest. But on reflection I have to say no, that is not the case. What I realize is that a number of different experiences led me in this direction. For example, my grandmothers each had a whole compendium of folk remedies that worked as well as any "patent" medicine for a variety of simple afflictions. We always turned first to these remedies. If they didn't work, then we would consult the health professionals in the family. Frankly, I always believed the grandmothers were more knowledgeable.

Then when I became a registered nurse, I encountered many cases where tried and true medical approaches just didn't work. Mostly these failures occurred with chronic conditions. After becoming a psychiatric clinical specialist working in community settings such as group homes and clinics, I realized that mental health problems are just one aspect of a much bigger societal picture and only one aspect of a person who is a spiritual, physical, social, and intellectual being. Just providing the right chemical support for the psychiatric condition does not address the societal issues or other aspects of the person.

Perhaps the biggest turning point for me, when I really internalized that there are many ways to define health and to bring about healing, was when I participated in a healing ceremony on the Navajo reservation. This experience rocked my scientific mindset and caused me to begin investigating other systems of healing with an open mind.

About this same time, my own health underwent a radical shift and conventional methods of treatment only partly solved the problem. Eventually, I settled on an integrated approach that includes yoga, massage, walking, and energy work on a regular basis along with conventional (allopathic) treatment. I am as healthy as a horse these days and attribute my well being to this integrated approach.

Lastly, I am both a nurse and a professional artist. For all of my professional life I have struggled with these twin loves. Over the course of the last decade, I have finally integrated these two seemingly disparate disciplines into a nursing practice and research agenda that focuses on the whole person. I express a person's biography in visual art. This process is described by participants as very healing even when they have medical conditions that cannot be solved. Through this process the person makes connections, uncovers important life patterns, identifies life symbols, and creates new meanings. This work has led me to question definitions of health and of healing and has prompted me to more closely examine the aesthetic aspects of healing work.

Q: Do you think CAM really works?

A: Well, yes and no. It depends on which CAM you are asking about and what you mean by "really work." Will every CAM cure a specific condition, even the condition it purports to cure? No. But do some unconventional, non-allopathic strategies promote, maintain, or restore health, even though current research methods have no way of demonstrating how they do this? Absolutely! And here is where I have to talk about the responsibility of each person to become informed about the efficacy of CAM they are considering learning about either for their own health or as a practitioner of the method or approach.

There are some CAM that have been well researched using accepted scientific approaches and have proven to be effective for certain conditions. Massage, acupuncture, yoga, certain herbal remedies, selected nutritional supplements and dietary approaches, and transcendental meditation are some of these. The important thing for a prospective user or practitioner is to investigate what has been studied before making a personal choice or before choosing a program. As a practitioner, it is absolutely a practical and ethical necessity to study what is known about the efficacy of certain CAM before recommending them to others. With so much information available on the Internet, many patients are more knowledgeable than practitioners. However, it is up to the practitioner to discriminate between information that has dubious origins or studies that lack scientific rigor of any sort. Many unsubstantiated claims are made for certain CAM.

Q: Are there any driving forces to include CAM in the education of nurses?

A: Yes, there are. First, consumers are asking for information and referrals to CAM. A landmark study in 1993 reported that one in three Americans use therapies or treatment approaches that are considered to be unconventional.[1] In a follow-up study by the same research team in 1997, it was found that over 629 million visits were made to alternative practitioners.[2] In the years between the two studies, the use of unconventional therapies increased 47%. In response to the growing interest by consumers, accrediting agencies are beginning to require the inclusion of content on CAM in nursing curricula. For example, *The Essentials of Baccalaureate Education* published by the American Association of Colleges of Nursing requires content on alternative and complementary therapies.[3] The majority of nursing programs (77%) include content related to CAM[4] compared to two-thirds of medical schools.[5] The White House Commission on Complementary and Alternative Medicine's recent final report suggests that conventional practitioners should be educated in complementary therapies, and vice versa.

Q: What are the issues regarding CAM in the education of health professionals?

A: Well, this is a complex question. In May of 2002, the *Online Journal in Nursing* published an article that I wrote about this topic relating to nursing education.[6] Although I was specifically addressing nursing education, the issues identified in this article remain true for the education of other health professionals as well. The major issue is curriculum development and design.

Before an educational program can be initiated, a curriculum must be developed. The curriculum is designed by the faculty taking into consideration the requirements of accrediting bodies, licensing requirements, practice acts, and other legal requirements. Regulation, standards of practice, curricula in other similar programs, clinical opportunities, amount and availability of research on efficacy of practitioners and practices, and concerns about demonstrating clinical competence are all issues to be addressed. Furthermore, the faculty must take into account the health needs of the population in the area of the educational program unless the program is a national one. In that case, national demographics must be considered rather than local ones. Then, there is the issue of faculty expertise and interest. These also figure into how the curriculum is designed.

To ensure the possibility of success, the faculty of any program must reach a philosophical consensus on certain key questions. What is the desired outcome of the program? Is it an educational program or a training program? If education is the goal, then more breadth, depth, and complexity are required. Is healing or curing the most acceptable outcome of care? What constitutes cure? Healing? Are people composites of parts or integrated wholes inseparable from the context of their lives?

The ways in which faculty addresses these concerns (and other similar questions) will drive the curriculum and influence the outcomes of the program. Faculty, even those with similar views, may have significant differences in philosophy that affect curriculum design. For example, the variations in philosophy in nursing programs can be quite extreme because of the breadth of the discipline. On any given faculty there may be those steeped in a reductionist view of science as well as those embracing a holistic (or New Science) view. Both paradigms have produced influential philosophers and theorists in nursing. Though one can take the position that these two paradigms are not mutually exclusive, that is a minority view. More frequently, differences rather than similarities are highlighted in philosophical discourse, making the development of a curriculum a difficult task indeed.

Q: How do you base the CAM curriculum on evidenced-based practice?

A: Curricula are based on research and prevailing practice. Research in CAM, although improving, still leaves much to be desired even if a broad definition of research is used. This is true because many of the phenomena supposedly involving CAM are either immeasurable using current technology or otherwise ineffable. Even more problematic is that there are CAM for which there are no national standards of practice and no core curriculum have been identified, making both regulation and curriculum development for these much more difficult.

Q: Is there a taxonomy across disciplines that is used in CAM ?

A: We have yet to settle on how to define and language CAM. "Traditional," "unconventional," "alternative," "complementary," and "integrated" are all terms used to denote the kinds of therapies we are discussing. Exactly what language we will settle on as a culture is still unclear. Schools for health professionals have to reach a consensus about the definition of these therapies. Language in this matter reflects philosophies, and sometimes reaching consensus about the language to use can be as thorny as reaching a more general philosophical consensus.

Q: How many courses related to CAM should be taught in a healthcare curriculum?

A: Well, first it is necessary to determine the desired outcome: an education program or a training program. For example, a training program for a specific skill is more abbreviated and has less breadth and depth than an education program and thus, requires fewer courses. Likewise, if the program is an education program and not a training program for a specific CAM, faculty also must take into account how much of the curriculum should be devoted to CAM. What percentage of the student's practice will involve the use of or referral to CAM? With every healthcare discipline almost exponentially increasing their body of knowledge, at some point there is more content than can possibly be taught. What is essential and what is simply desirable?

Q: Are there ethical issues related to CAM and education?

A: Yes, there are ethical considerations. For example, when there is no sound research evidence to suggest the therapeutic value of a CAM, it is not hard to dismiss it. But what about those cases where the research results in conflicting data? Also, some CAM are based on worldviews that challenge that of the dominant culture and thus, the majority of educators in the health professions. For example, those therapies involving subtle energies of the body have been particularly maligned as in conflict with Christian values. Both faculty and students may be ethically uncomfortable with including content that challenges prevailing values and beliefs which may seem to be morally questionable.

Q: How do healthcare providers claim "competency" in their practice?

A: The issue of competency is an ethical issue as well as a practice issue. If there are no regulations (or if regulations vary dramatically from state to state), no national standards of practice, and no core curriculum for a CAM, should a health professional use it or refer to it? What is the legal liability of using or referring to such a practice, especially for practitioners who are licensed (such as nurses, physicians, and other allied health professionals)? And what about quality assurance in such cases? At the very least, licensed providers must be aware of the required qualifications of CAM practitioners and the type of training they receive. Nurses employing CAM must ensure that they have proof of their qualifications (i.e., certificates, certifications), that the practice does not violate the state's Nurse Practice Act, that they adhere to nursing's Code of Ethics, and that they carry proper insurance.

Q: What are other issues related to clinical practice?

A: Where will students practice CAM skills if there are few practitioners in the area and if these therapies are not accepted in practice settings? Students need role models and settings in which to learn and practice new skills. Educators are obligated to create curricula that account for these learning needs.

Q: What is the relationship between holistic nursing, CAM, and integrative practice?

A: This is a very interesting question that takes me back to the issues of paradigms and language. Holistic nursing is a philosophy. It is also a growing subspecialty in nursing. It is somewhat distressing that a philosophy first given voice by the founder of modern secular nursing, Florence Nightingale, should not be the reality in every school of nursing. Although holism is often given "lip service" in the philosophies of nursing schools, it is not actually embraced by the majority of schools. This is in spite of the fact that at least six prominent nursing theorists and philosophers support such a basis for both education and practice. The reasons for this are many and varied and I won't address them here. However, the American Holistic Nurses' Association was founded to address the need for more holistic practice based on a worldview that challenges the prevailing nursing paradigm. The old paradigm is changing toward a more holistic view, albeit slowly. Perhaps at some point there will be no need to discriminate holistic nursing as a specialty because it will be part and parcel of every curriculum and even tested in National Boards.

In some minds holistic nursing is defined as the use of CAM in nursing practice. Although many holistic nurses embrace certain CAM, the use of these does not identify a nurse as holistic. The reason that the use of CAM and holistic nursing has been so closely linked is that many CAM are based on a worldview that is holistic. Holistic thinking and belief is the common ground.

"Integrative practice" is a fairly new term in nursing and refers to one which is holistic in philosophy and inclusive in terms of therapeutic approaches. The American Holistic Nurses' Association Standards of Advanced Holistic Nursing Practice for Graduate-Prepared Nurses defines integrative as a patient- and relationship-centered approach to care that incorporates complementary and conventional services and interventions.

In summary, it seems to me that "integrative" refers to "how" holistic nurses could practice to include conventional and unconventional approaches to care and at the advanced practice level to help in differential diagnosis, treatment, and care.

Q: Are there standards of practice to guide nurses in using CAM?

A: Happily, I can say a resounding "yes" to this question. The American Holistic Nurses' Association has provided the leadership, the forum, and the support to develop these standards for both basic and advanced practice. The process of standards developed took several years, involved many experts in education, practice, and research and was based on research. Participating in the process as the National Task Force Chair for the standards for graduate prepared nurses has given me a unique opportunity to appreciate both the complexity and the value of standards development. Any group seeking to gain credibility in practice needs to create standards of practice based on both research and prevailing practices. Standards can then be used to develop a core curriculum. From the core curriculum, education or training programs can be developed, as well as a test, to insure minimum levels of competency. This process of standards development, core curriculum development, and certification development is one that if used really does help to insure quality in care.

Q: What guidelines are available regarding curriculum development and CAM?

A: As mentioned, The American Holistic Nurses' Association (ANHA) has published a Core Curriculum for holistic nursing. Barbara Dossey provided the leadership for the development of the first curriculum. At this point, given that there are new standards for both basic and advanced nursing, it is necessary to revisit the core curriculum and revise it. This revision should reflect the enormous changes that are taking place in the whole areas of CAM and the mandate by the Office of Alternative Medicine and others to include such content in nursing (and medical) programs. This curriculum could be a guide to schools of nursing as educators make changes to include

CAM content. Currently, I am chair of the national task force to develop a national core curriculum for holistic nurses. Naturally, such a curriculum will address the issue of CAM content.

Inclusion of CAM content in nursing education has been uneven. Mary Fenton and others are working to provide data on exactly which colleges of nursing are including CAM and what kind of content they are including.[7] We are eagerly awaiting the results of their study. At this point, we can be sure there is a great deal of disparity in content regarding CAM among colleges of nursing.

At the AHNA national conventions in 1998 and 2002, educators in holistic nursing met to discuss educational issues and needs. At the upcoming pre-convention workshops we will be meeting again and discussing curriculum needs and approaches to curriculum design and content.

Q: What is the difference between a certificate and certification in CAM?

A: This is an extremely important question. The terms "certificate," "certification," and "licensure" are frequently used very imprecisely, but their precise meanings are especially important when it comes to discussing CAM.

A certificate is issued to demonstrate that a learner has completed a course of study that is not associated with an academic degree. Anyone can issue one although certificates that are to be used as proof of continuing education in both nursing and medicine require that programs meet specific criteria.

A certification recognizes excellence in practice and is issued by organizations in the discipline. The first field in nursing to establish certification was the National Association of Nurse Anesthetists in 1946. In 1955 nurse midwives began to get certified. Certification programs in nursing have proliferated. Certification began as a voluntary effort to establish competency and credibility in nursing specialties by the organizations representing those agencies. State regulatory agencies are not involved in certification; however, some state nurse practice acts now include requirements for certification for nurses to practice in advanced roles. The American Nursing Credentialing Center is the largest certifying body in nursing. However, some specialties such a holistic nursing have their own certification boards. I have been a member of the American Holistic Nurses' Certification Corporation Board which provides a certification process that allows nurses wishing to establish their credibility in this area of nursing at either the basic or advanced levels.

It is very important to recognize that certification is NOT licensure. In the healthcare profession, licensure is based on a practice act, a piece of legislation in each state that defines the practice of the field. Licensure essentially demonstrates to the public that a person has met the minimum requirements to hold a license, usually proof of graduation from an accredited program and passing scores on board exams. In nursing these exams are national. Licensure is a regulatory practice that defines the length of time a license is valid, requirements for renewal, and provisions for revoking the license. To further ensure safe practice, practice acts designate a regulatory board. The regulatory boards administer the practice act. In most cases, membership on State Boards of Nursing are governor appointments.

Q: How does CAM relate to theories of nursing?

A: There are several nurse theorists whose worldview is holistic. Therefore, their theories can provide guidance to nurses seeking to practice using a solid theoretical base and who want to include CAM in their practices. Martha Rogers, Jean Watson, Rosemarie Parse, Margaret Newman, Callista Roy (in her later writings especially), and Helen Erickson are examples of theorists that offer a solid theoretical foundation for holistic nursing practice. Standards for both basic and advanced practice in holistic nursing require that practice be theory-based.

Theory in any field is the basis for understanding the discipline. In practice, disciplines having a clear theoretical basis provides a language, a basis for inquiry, credibility, intellectual satisfaction, and a more satisfying practice. One of the problematic issues in CAM is that many of the theories that are the basis of practice are in question due to a paucity of research demonstrating the viability of the theory. The theory, research, practice circle is one that just can't be ignored or the body of knowledge in the field will become irrelevant as our understanding of human beings, health, and healing change. Scholarship in any discipline is the bedrock of safe and effective practice.

An important framework for knowledge development in nursing may serve other disciplines and CAM practitioners as they seek to develop the body of knowledge regarding CAM. In 1978, Barbara Carper, then a graduate student at Texas Women's University, surveyed nursing literature and identified four fundamental patterns of knowing in nursing.[8] She categorized these patterns of knowing as empirical, ethical, personal, and esthetic. Empirical knowing relates to objective, publicly verifiable knowledge. What we know in this category can be quantified and measured. Ethical knowing related to the necessity of moral insight in nursing (and indeed in any human science). It examines various ethical philosophies and approaches to decision making. Personal knowing refers to the necessary self awareness that nurses must have to create effective interpersonal relationships with both patients and colleagues. Esthetic knowing refers to the art of nursing, the way in which nursing is enacted, and the beauty in these acts of the nurse. This framework might be a useful starting point for practitioners to think about in developing the body of knowledge in any healthcare field. Chinn and Kramer[9] have proposed that integrated knowledge development in nursing could be accomplished using this model.

Q: What would you recommend to colleges of nursing that are considering the inclusion of CAM content?

A: Educators might find it useful to consult the American Holistic Nurses' Association core curriculum, the Office of Alternative Medicine, and various journals that include CAM content such as *The Journal of Holistic Nursing*, *Alternative Therapies*, and *Holistic Nursing Practice*. The American Holistic Nurses' *Association Standards of Advanced Holistic Nursing Practice for Graduate-Prepared Nurses* clearly delineates practice expectations regarding CAM in the Section "Core Value Five: The Holistic Caring Process."

I would also recommend the article I wrote for *The Online Journal in Nursing*.[6] It identifies some of the pitfalls that faculty can encounter and offers solutions or examples of how others have met these challenges.

Suggested Readings

Erickson HC, Tomlin E, Swain, MW. *Modeling and Role Modeling: A Theory and Paradigm for Nursing.* Lexington, SC: Pine Press; 1984.

Picard C, Jones DA, eds. *Giving Voice to What We Know: Margaret Neuman's Theory of Health as Expanding Conciousness in Practice, Research, and Education.* Sudbury, MA: Jones and Bartlett Publishers; 2005.

Parse R. Illuminations: *The Human Becoming Theory in Practice and Research.* Sudbury, MA: Jones and Bartlett Publishers; 1999.

Rogers, ME. Science of unitary human beings. In: Malinski VM, ed. *Exploration on Martha Rogers Science of Unitary Human Beings.* Norwalk, CTB: Appleton-Century-Crafts; 1986.

Barnes, B. *Roy Adaptation Model-Based Research: 25 Years of Contributions to Nursing Science.* Indianapolis, IN: Center Nursing Press, 1999.

Watson, J. *Caring Science as Sacred Science.* Philadelphia, PA: F.A. Davis Company; 2004.

References

1. Eisenberg D, Kessler R, Foster C, Norlock F, Calkins D, Delbanco T. Unconventional medicine in the United States: prevalance, costs, and patterns of use. *N Eng J Med.* 2001;328(4):246–252.

2. Eisenberg D, Davis R, Ettner S, Appel S, Wilkey S., Van Rompay M, Kessler RC. Trends in alternative medicine use in the United States, 1990–1997: results of a follow-up national survey. *JAMA.* 1998;280(18):1569–1575.

3. American Association of Colleges of Nursing. *Essentials of Baccelaureate Education for Professional Nursing Practice.* Washington, DC; 1998.

4. Richardson S. Complementary health and healing in nursing education. *J Holistic Nursing.* 2003;21(1):20–35.

5. Chez R, Jonas W, Crawford C. (2001) A survey of medical students opinion about complementary and alternative medicine. *Am J Obst Gynecol.* 2001;185(3): 754–757.

6. Gaydos HL. Complementary and alternative therapies in nursing education: trends and issues. *Online J Issues Nurs.* 2001;6(2):5.

7. Fenton MV, Morris D. The integration of holistic nursing practices and complementary and alternative modalities into curricula of schools of nursing. *Altern Ther Health Med.* 2003;9(4):62–67.

8. Carper B. Fundamental patterns of knowing in nursing. *Adv Nurs Sci.* 1978;10(1): 13–23.

9. Chinn P, Kramer, MK. *Integrated Knowledge Development in Nursing.* 6th ed. St. Louis, MO: Mosby; 2004.

6

Traditional Chinese Medicine (TCM)

William A. Berno, AP

About the Author

William A. Berno graduated from Quantum University's Homeopathic Program and is a diplomate of the National Board of Homeopathic Examiners. He has been teaching acupuncture and homeopathy for the last five years and has a private practice in Sarasota and Clearwater, Florida. He is also a teacher of Transcendental Meditation and has been practicing this technique for the past 36 years. Dr. Berno holds a Bachelor of Arts in English from the University of South Florida and a Master of Fine Arts from the University of California, San Diego.

Q: Tell me about your background in Traditional Chinese Medicine (TCM). What got you interested in this approach as a physician?

A: I come from a medical family. There are many RNs in my family: my father, mother, sister, aunt, niece, and grandmother. My father and mother owned a nursing home in Florida. My grandfather and uncle were MDs and two uncles were dentists. So I know the inside story of Western medicine, also referred to as conventional and allopathic medicine. Every time I sneezed or my gums bled I received a shot of penicillin. I was always interested in helping people, but the subtle energetic approach to healing always appealed to me. In my 20s I started visiting chiropractors and acupuncturists. I decided to pursue the Eastern approach to healing because if offered me a way to be of service to people in a wholistic manner. With a license in acupuncture, I could incorporate many different modalities on my healing menu: acupuncture, homeopathy, Moxibustion (burning the herb Mugwort on or near the needle for circulation and healing purposes), medicinal herbs, Tui Na (Chinese massage), and other forms of healing energy such as Medical Qi Gong and Reiki.

Q: What is TCM and what are its roots?

A: The roots of TCM go back 4000 to 10,000 years in the "New Stone Age." Needles made of stone, called bian needles, were found from this period by archeologists. Bian needles were believed to be used for minute blood letting and regulating Qi circulation. Qi, as explained in ancient Chinese philosophy is the fundamental substance constituting the Universe. Everything is different manifestations of this energy force called Qi. In the Shang Dynasty of 3000 years ago, hieroglyphics of acupuncture and Moxibustion appeared in the inscriptions on bones and tortoise shells.

Q: What are the fundamental principles of TCM?

A: The fundamental principles of TCM are the theory of Yin and Yang (night and day, cold and hot, etc.), the Five Elements (fire, earth, metal, water, wood), the 12 major meridians that correspond to the major organs of the body (heart, spleen, lungs, kidneys and liver, etc.) and the Pathogenic Factors (wind, cold, summer-heat, dampness, dryness, and fire).

Q: What does Yin and Yang have to do with TCM?

A: The concept of Yin and Yang is first referenced in the "Book of Changes," dating back to about 1000 to 770 BC. It is believed that Yin and Yang was derived from the peasants' observation of the cyclical alternation of day and night. Day is Yang and night is Yin. This dualistic approach in interpreting nature was to use nature's laws in a positive way and not trying to control or subdue nature as is found in many conventional medical approaches. The beauty of the Yin and Yang approach is that it is not stagnant. Yang moves into Yin and Yin into Yang. They are in opposition but are also interdependent. In the medical practice of TCM a simple Yin/Yang treatment principle would be if the patient is too Yin (cold) we would tonify (strengthen) his or her Yang (fire) aspect to bring a balance to the physical environment.

Q: What part does the theory of Five Elements have to do in TCM diagnosis?

A: The theory of Five Elements came after the concept of Yin and Yang. It was first referenced about 476–221 BC during the Warring States Period. The Five Elements are wood, fire, earth, metal, and water. Each refers to two organs and many other aspects such as emotions, colors, tastes, sense organs, tissues, sounds, etc. The Five Elements generate each other, they control each other, they overact on each other, and sometimes insult each other. For example, wood is liver/gall bladder, the emotion is anger, the sound is shouting, the color is green, the season is Spring, the taste is sour and wood opens into the eyes. Wood generates fire (wood burns), overacts on Earth (roots), and is controlled by metal (ax).

Q: What modalities of healing therapy does TCM encompass?

A: The healing therapies that TCM encompasses are Tui Na (Chinese Massage), Moxibustion (burning of the herb Mugwort on or near the needle), electrical stimulation on the needles generating a "tapping" feeling and making the treatment stronger, herbal preparations in raw or patent form, Qi Gong (which is energy stimulation from the practitioner to the needle or patient), and of course different needling techniques with stainless steel needles.

Q: What is Medical Qi Gong?

A: As stated earlier, Qi is the fundamental substance constituting the Universe. Everything is different manifestations of this energy force called Qi. All vital activities of the human body are explained by changes and movement of Qi. When Qi does not move, TCM calls this pain stagnation of Qi. When there is lassitude, TCM calls this deficiency of Qi. These pathologies can be expressed both on the physical as well as mental or emotional aspects of one's life. Qi means energy; Gong means force. Medical Qi Gong is a technique where by the practitioner activates his or her own Qi energy and transfers this vital force to the patient via the needles or directly to the body. It can be physically felt. Qi Gong masters can transfer high voltage electrical shocks to their patients. A practitioner must have a strong nervous system to practice Medical Qi Gong.

Q: How does TCM diagnose a patient?

A: TCM diagnoses a patient in many ways. It is accomplished by simply looking at all aspects of the patient:
- The way he or she walks, stands, and sits;
- Observing his or her Shen (the "Spirit" of the face and eyes);
- Hearing the sound of the patient's voice, the heart, the lungs;
- Smelling the odor of the patient;
- Asking questions of the patient;
- Touching the patient by taking the 12 pulses;
- Diagnosing the abdomen;
- Temperature and texture of the skin; and
- Palpating the meridians of the body.

Q: What part does the 8 Principle Diagnosis play in TCM?

A: Eight Principle Diagnosis in TCM encompasses all other aspects of diagnosis. It is all-inclusive. It incorporates Channel Theory, Organ Theory, and Yin/Yang Theory. The 8 Principles are Interior/Exterior, Hot/Cold, Excess/Deficient, and Yin/Yang. Eight Principle Diagnosis is not to pigeonhole a pathology; it is to unravel complicated patterns and identify their basic contradictions so the physician can arrive at a treatment protocol that is focused on the most relevant aspect of the case. If a patient presents with burning in the epigastrium, bleeding gums, thirst, insomnia, red tongue, and full-rapid pulse this would be diagnosed in 8 Principles as Excess-Heat in the stomach (interior).

Q: What are the benefits of using TCM in combination with conventional therapies?

A: Acupuncture, per se, does 3 basic things:
1. When the needle is in the acupuncture point, it brings more blood circulation to the area, causing more white blood cells to carry away toxins and red blood cells to strengthen the healing process;
2. The acupuncture needle in the correct point breaks up the stagnation, allowing the Qi to flow and relieving pain in that area, as pain in TCM is stagnant Qi;
3. When the needle is inserted into the acupuncture point it has been found by conventional medicine that the natural pain killers of the body, the beta endorphins, are naturally and spontaneously released causing a relaxation and well-being response for the patient.

The benefits of using TCM in combination with conventional therapies is that TCM can bring the healing process to fruition more quickly with less use of toxic drugs and invasive therapies. The hospitals in China have a wing for acupuncture, for surgery and Western treatment, for herbs, Qi Gong, and Tui Na (Chinese massage).

Q: Is there clinical evidence that TCM works?

A: In the *American Journal of Acupuncture,* **www.acupuncturejournal.com**, a person can find many documented clinical studies on acupuncture. For example, Sumano and Mateos[1] presented studies on wound healing with acupuncture (including before and after pictures). In the same publication, Elgert and Omsted[2] report a case of a 17-year-old female diagnosed with chronic inflammatory demyelinating polyradiculoneuropathy (CIDP), a rare neruological disease characterized by progressive symmetrical motor and sensory loss. The current biomedical treatments are reported as limited; however, the young lady was treated successfully with acupuncture. In the same issue there is a report of varicose veins successfully treated with acupuncture[3] and a comparative study on the treatment of migraine headache using acupuncture versus conventional drug therapy.[4]

While there is a multitude of research in acupuncture, many of the designs have not been of the highest quality due to sample size, randomization, or sham procedures. However, research continues to show promise as stuides are now examining the mechanism of action through diagnostic measurements. Positive outcomes have been seen in nausea and vomiting in chemotherapy, dental pain, headache, menstrual cramps, fibromyalgia,[5] osteoarthritis,[6] and back pain.[7]

Q: What can be done to encourage the acceptance of TCM in conventional medical practices?

A: Experience is the best teacher. Intellectual arguments are a waste of time. Conventional Western medical doctors should have the personal experience of acupuncture, and acupuncturists should be invited into the hospital setting to show how these two disciples can work together to bring quicker and more profound relief for patients.

Q: How are medical students and other healthcare students educated in relation to TCM?

A: Major medical facilities such as Harvard Medical School have students studying major acupuncture meridians along with their regular physiology. The University of Virginia is incorporating complimentary and alternative therapies in their curriculum for medical students.

Q: How are hospitals using TCM in health care now?

A: A clinic in Seattle integrates Eastern and Western medicine in regular patient care. I personally worked with a psychiatrist in Clearwater, Florida. He referred many patients for acupuncture and he reported that their psychiatric sessions went much better after receiving regular acupuncture treatment.

There is definitely a movement toward integrating alternative therapies and Eastern medical protocols with traditional allopathic therapies in major hospitals through patient education. At Sarasota Memorial Hospital in Sarasota, FL, upon request of patients, acupuncturists have been allowed to come into the hospital to give treatments to their patients. I personally know that at Sarasota Memorial, nurses are allowed to give Reiki treatments to patients.

Q: How can we break down the barriers that conventional medical practices have in relation to CAM?

A: We have to find Western MDs who are open to CAM. We have to infiltrate through their ranks. We have to make believers of them. As I said before, experience is the best teacher. We have to have dialogues and see if there are possibilities to work together. I also think the issues of finance need to be addressed because I believe this is one of the biggest barriers to successful cooperation. I know several MDs who use alternative therapies in Sarasota. We have to start where we can be heard.

Suggested Readings

American College of TCM. Available at: http://www.actcm.org/

Qi Journal Home Page. Available at: http://www.qi-journal.com/

Traditional Chinese Medicine and Qigong. Traditional Chinese Medicine. Available at: http://www.index-china.com/index-english/TCM-s.html. Accessed October 28, 2005.

Kaptchuk T. *The Web That Has No Weaver: Understanding Chinese Medicine.* New York, NY: Contemporary Books; 2000.

Beinfield H, Korngold E. *Between Heaven and Earth.* New York, NY: Ballantine Books; 1992.

Tierra M, Tierra L. *Chinese Traditional Herbal Medicine.* Vol. 1: Diagnosis and Treatment. Twin Lakes, WI: Lotus Press; 1998.

References

1. Sumano H, Mateos G. The use of acupuncture-like electrical stimulation for wound healing of lesions unresponsive to conventional treatement. *Am J Acupunct.* 1999;27(1–2):15–21.

2. Elgert G, Olmsted L. The treatment of chronic inflammatory demyelinating polyradiculoneuropathy with acupuncture: a clinical case study. *Am J Acupunct.* 1999;27(1–2):15–21.

3. Bodenheim R. Case report: successful treatment of varicose veins with acupuncture. *Am J Acupunct.* 1999;27(1–2):23–25.

4. Gao S, Zhao D, Xie Y. A comparative study on the treatment of migraine headache with combined distant and local acupuncture points versus conventional drug therapy. *Am J Acupunct.* 1999;27(1–2):27–30.

5. Assefi NP, Sherman KJ, Jacobsen C, Goldberg J, Smith WR, Buchwald D. A randomized clinical trial of acupuncture compared with sham acupuncture in fibromyalgia. [summary for patients in Ann Intern Med. 2005 Jul 5;143(1):I24;PMID: 1599874]. *Annals of Internal Medicine.* Jul 5 2005;143(1):10–19.

6. Vas J, Mendez C, Perea-Milla E, et al. Acupuncture as a complementary therapy to the pharmacological treatment of osteoarthritis of the knee: randomized controlled trial. *BMJ.* Nov 20 2004;329(7476):1216.

7. Furlan AD, van Tulder MW, Cherkin DC, et al. Acupuncture and dry needling for low back pain. [update of Cochrane Database Syst Rev. 2002;(2)CD001351; PMID 107963434]. *Cochrane Database of Systematic Reviews.* 2005(1):CD001351.

7

Ayurveda

Vasant Lad, MASc

About the Author

Vasant Lad is a native of India who has been a practitioner and professor of Ayurvedic medicine for more than 20 years and is considered to be one of the world's foremost experts in Ayurveda. He holds a Bachelor of Ayurvedic Medicine & Surgery (BAMS), a Master of Ayurvedic Science (MASc), and his academic and practical training includes the study of allopathic medicine (Western medicine). He served as medical director of the Ayurveda Hospital in Pune, India, for three years and held the position of professor of clinical medicine for 12 years. He is the founder and director of the Ayurvedic Institute in Albuquerque, New Mexico. Since 1984, he has conducted one of the first full-time programs of Ayurveda study in the United States. Dr. Lad is the author of *Ayurveda: The Science of Self-Healing*.

Q: How did you get interested in Ayurveda?

A: That's a very interesting story. When I was a schoolboy, my grandma, who was in her late 80s, had renal failure. She was dying. The doctors said there was no medicine for her other than steroids and antibiotics. I witnessed this suffering pretty closely. At that time my father had a close friend, Dr. Mama Gohklae, who was an Ayurvedic doctor. He came to our home and saw my grandma. She had such swelling all over her body that it was difficult to feel her pulse. He felt it at the root of her thumb. For about ten minutes he felt her pulse and wrote things down. He looked into her eyes, at her tongue, and noted the swelling all over her body. He made an Ayurvedic herbal formula and he asked me to administer it to my grandma, as I had such affection and love for her. So, I would make the herbal tea and herbal concoctions and give it to my grandma. There were also certain diet restrictions. The amazing thing is that within two weeks her swelling had gone away, her blood pressure came back to normal, and her health improved. So, my father's close friend, Dr. Mama Gohklae, and my father both inspired me to learn Ayurveda.

Q: How were you educated and trained in Ayurveda?

A: At that time there was an integrated Ayurvedic medical college. Pune University had parallel courses in Ayurvedic and allopathic training, called Integrated Ayurvedic Medical Courses. The degree they granted was a BAMS, a Bachelor of Ayurvedic Medicine and Surgery. So, I was a student at Tilak Ayurveda Mahavidyalaya and learned both allopathic medicine and Ayurvedic medicine, allopathic, modern anatomy and Ayurvedic anatomy, modern physiology and Ayurvedic physiology, modern psychology and Ayurvedic psychology. We had highly trained medical doctors who gave lectures on modern medicine. Similarly, Ayurvedic physicians (vaidyas) gave lectures on the same topic, but from an Ayurvedic perspective. In that way I learned an integrated approach that included both Ayurvedic and modern medicine. I saw the beauty of both sciences. Every science has its right place in the field of healing.

Q: Was integrated medicine popular at that time?

A: Oh, at that time it was very popular.

Q: In your classical medical school education, at what point did they start having you go into the hospital and begin working with patients?

A: Every program module of classes was actually 18 months long. In the first module we learned principles and philosophy of both Ayurvedic and modern medicine. In the second module, students would join the hospital and there Ayurvedic doctors and modern doctors would teach us how to read pulse, how to check blood pressure, how to examine the patient, and how to administer medicine. We started our clinical studies in the second module. There were three modules totaling four and a half years of study. Then I did a two-year internship working in the hospital. During the internship I worked in every department of Ayurveda: pediatrics, geriatrics, internal medicine, surgery, gynecology, obstetrics, and ENT (ear, nose, and throat).

Q: **After you graduated from Ayurvedic medical school what did you do?**

A: To have some income during my internship, I became a lecturer and started giving lectures on Ayurvedic nidana panchaka (the classical five barometers of etiology and pathology). From my experience as a lecturer, I became a junior professor. I spent about 15 years teaching Ayurveda and practicing Ayurveda simultaneously. As an instructor, I progressed through the levels of the college becoming a senior professor, an examiner, and eventually a postgraduate examiner.

Our institute was affiliated with Pune University, a full-fledged medical school with a 200-bed medical hospital. We practiced Ayurvedic and modern surgeries, Ayurvedic medicine, and modern medicine. It was wonderful training for me; I obtained both theoretical and practical knowledge of Ayurveda by teaching and practicing at the hospital. I also started my own clinic about 10 miles east of Pune and went there in the evenings. The whole day I was working and in the evenings I would go and treat the village people, the poor people. Like a barefooted doctor, I would walk with my briefcase or ride my bicycle and go door-to-door, examining the patients and helping the poor people. So after graduating from Ayurveda Medical College, I lectured at Tilak Ayurveda Mahavidyalaya, worked in the Ayurvedic hospital there, and had my own private practice.

Q: **If somebody asked you what Ayurveda is, what would you say? What are the eight classical branches?**

A: The Sanskrit word "Ayurveda" is derived from two words, "ayu" which means life, and "veda" which means knowledge. Ayurveda is the knowledge of life, and knowledge that is systematized becomes science, so Ayurveda became the "science of life." As I studied Ayurveda in depth, I saw that it is not only a medicine, but it is a complete way of living life in harmony with nature, creating balance between body, mind, and consciousness. According to Ayurveda, every individual is a unique expression of cosmic consciousness. Every individual is a distinct phenomenon and every individual has a unique body type, which is called "prakruti," the individual constitution. There are five elements that combine in pairs to form three interactions or doshas. Each element is associated with senses: ether with learning, air with touch, fire with vision, water with taste, and earth with smell. Due to changing seasons, changing diet, lifestyle, emotional changes, and changes in relationship, three dosha bodily organizations called "vata" (air and ether), "pitta" (fire and water), and "kapha" (water and earth) undergo change. This altered state of the dosha is called "vikruti." Though vikruti is not a disease, it can create a potential space for future disorders. Ayurveda looks at every individual through the prakruti/vikruti paradigm. These branches of Ayurveda literally heal the person in all departments of life. These are the eight branches of Ayurveda:

1. Ayurveda medicine
2. surgery
3. gynecology
4. obstetrics and delivering the child
5. dentistry
6. ear, nose, and throat
7. Ayurveda geriatrics
8. spiritual or psychiatric therapy

Ayurveda gives us daily routines, seasonal routines, and personal routines so that we can keep balance in the bodily doshas. We can live in harmony with nature with proper diet and lifestyle, and through "panchakarma" (detoxification) and rejuvenation programs.

Q: What are the basic concepts of Ayurveda, such as constitution and imbalance as well as cause and effect? Could you just say a bit about the emphasis in Ayurveda on cause and effect?

A: Ayurvedic philosophy is based upon Sankhya philosophy. "Sankhya" means self realization. According to Sankhya's philosophy there exists Purusha, the conscious principle, and Prakruti, the primordial matter. The Universe is made up of a cause and effect phenomenon; "as the cause, so the effect." Cause is a conceived effect; effect is a revealed cause. So, behind every creation there is a cause that is called primordial prakruti. Similarly, behind the creation of each human being there is a cause, which is individual prakruti and an effect, which is vikruti. In fact, cause and effect is such an intimate phenomenon that every disease has a cause, every illness has a cause, every disorder has a cause, and every suffering has a definite cause. One of the skills of an Ayurvedic physician is discovering the etiological factors that have occurred in that particular patient. It could be any number of things such as incorrect diet, wrong lifestyle, imbalanced emotional background, or even repressed emotions. Even judgment or criticism can be the cause that affects the bodily dosha.

If the cause is kapha provoking—such as dairy products, cheese, yogurt, cold drinks, sleeping during the day, and a sedentary lifestyle—it will increase kapha. Hot, spicy foods, working in the hot sun, and emotions such as anger, hate, envy, or jealousy will aggravate pitta. Causes that increase vata include eating old food or leftover food, raw vegetables, doing physical exercise constantly, working too hard, and emotions such as fear, insecurity, and loneliness. These causes will lead to disease that reflects the imbalanced dosha—vata, pitta, or kapha. The phenomenon of cause and effect is a basic condition of Sankhya's philosophy and Ayurveda, in principle and practice, has totally accepted that.

Q: What is the history of Ayurveda?

A: The history of Ayurveda is quite ancient, more than 5000 years old. Legend says that Brahma, the Creator, simply remembered Ayurveda. The root of Ayurvedic philosophy and Ayurvedic systems is in the Rig Veda. The ancient Vedic literatures are considered an authentic spiritual record. The Vedas unfolded in the heart of enlightened people. Whatever experience they brought forth through deep meditation, they verbally expressed to their students and the students remembered the teachings. Then later they recorded those teachings on palm leaves as Vedic spiritual scripture. These original scriptures still exist today and trace their origins back more than 10,000 years through this oral tradition. Another interesting thing to remember is that in ancient times the lifespan was much longer than it is today. There were some rishis (seers) who were hundreds, even thousands, of years old.

In this tradition, as I mentioned earlier, Brahma the creator remembered Ayurveda, then he told it to Prajapati. Prajapati then explained it to the Ashwin twin brothers, and the Ashwins explained it to the rishi (a sage or wise man), Agnivesha. Agnivesha explained it to Charaka. This knowledge was passed down in this way through the ages from the guru, the enlightened master, to his disciple and the disciple would accumulate and store it. The Charaka Samhita ("Samhita" means "collection") is an authentic record collected by Charaka's eight students into one work, the Charaka Samhita.

Q: From the beginning, any the enlightened rishis that perceived the knowledge of Ayurveda became teachers and taught their students, were each of these teachers and students Ayurvedic physicians in their own right?

A: The teacher would impart this knowledge to the disciple and then he would test him. He would ask questions and give certain information and instructions to test the student. When they had demonstrated their knowledge to the guru, he would tell them to practice and to go ahead and spread this knowledge. The teachers were physicians as well.

Q: How is Ayurveda relevant in today's world?

A: Ayurveda is quite relevant in today's world. In these days of modern technology with highly technical medicines, transplant surgery, laser beam surgery and genetic manipulation, modern medicine is moving so fast that they are overlooking the individual. Ayurveda encourages research and inquiry, but not at the expense of the individual. This is a crucial point: Ayurveda teaches us how to understand an individual; how to balance an individual; and how to create harmony between the body, mind, and consciousness in the daily life of the individual. Additionally, Ayurveda not only suggests medicines, but it gives us diet, lifestyle, cleansing, detoxification, and rejuvenation programs. All of this is quite relevant in today's world. A person may go to the doctor or the hospital, and have a variety of lab tests that indicate the person is normal. However, the person may still have pain, a coated tongue, headaches, and no happiness in their life. Ayurveda can help create balance, returning each individual to their healthy, happy, balanced state.

Q: What is the Ayurvedic definition of life?

A: The ancient texts say that life is the inseparable union of body, mind, and consciousness. Life is eternity. Life is timeless and life is living together with body, mind, and consciousness. Another text says life is constantly moving and changing. It is a current, a stream, a flow of experiencing, of looking, listening, learning, and living. Our concept of life is what we know only in the time interval between birth and death. But Ayurveda says there is life before birth, there is life between birth and death, and there is life after death. Life is eternally moving, changing, and transforming the energy field of consciousness and body and mind.

Q: How is health defined in Ayurveda?

A: According to Ayurveda, every individual has a unique constitution and every constitution has definite components of the constitution. These components of the constitution are the three doshas called vata (air and ether), pitta (fire and water), and kapha (water and earth); the seven dhatus (bodily tissues) called rasa (plasma), rakta (red blood cells), mamsa (muscles), meda (fat), asthi (bones), majja (nerves), and shukra (reproductive tissue); the three malas (bodily wastes) called mutra (urine), purisa (feces), and sweda (sweat); and the senses (ether, air, fire, water, and earth). This is what makes up an individual. Now, according to Ayurveda, every individual has a unique body type and every individual has a unique agni type. Agni is the gastric fire, or metabolic fire, which governs digestion, absorption, assimilation, and transformation of food into consciousness, into energy. According to Ayurveda, health is defined as a balance of the three doshas and one's agni or metabolic fire. Body weight is a criterion of determining constitutional, metabolic rate and is balanced when there is not much fluctuation of weight. Additionally, the seven bodily tissues should be in balance as well as the bodily wastes; no diarrhea or constipation, no polyuria or anuria. Ayurveda defines health as a state of balance between the three doshas, seven bodily tissues, three bodily wastes, and having a balanced state of mind and perception. Such a person will maintain a state of inner happiness, inner joy, and inner bliss. That is the definition of health in Ayurveda.

Q: What is the Ayurvedic concept of disease?

A: Ayurveda defines disease as to the result of wrong diet, improper lifestyle, emotional changes, and seasonal changes. Our bodily doshas are constantly changing in order to face those changes. There are 20 universal qualities (gunas), which are 10 pairs of opposites. They are present in the universe and they are present within the individual. Ayurveda is not only a biochemical science; it is a science of qualities, of the gunas. Our diet, lifestyle, emotional, and environmental changes are affected by those qualities in varying degrees. Suppose cold attracts cold. If a person has cold drinks and cold food during the cold season, the cold quality will be increased in the body—both the cold quality of kapha and the cold quality of vata. If the person has a vata prakruti, the result of this increase will be pain in the joints and stiffness in the muscles. If a person has a kapha-predominant prakruti, he might get a cold, congestion, or cough. Outer changes are constantly reacted to by inner biological changes. External ecology is constantly changing the internal ecology and these internal ecological changes are responsible for creating disease. Disease is aggravated dosha entering one or more of the seven bodily tissues, which first creates functional changes in the tissue, eventually causing structural changes in the affected tissue. These altered, modified functional and structural changes within the body/mind consciousness are disease. Another way to say this is that disease is the biochemical changes created within the tissue by aggravated dosha, which will affect both the function and structure of the tissue, organ, or system. That is what disease is.

Q: Could one say that imbalance precedes disease and if one could identify imbalance and rebalance that, one could prevent disease from occurring?

A: Yes. The imbalance can be revealed through psychosomatic symptomatology. Ayurveda uses clinical barometers to measure this. When an imbalance is quantified and qualified, it can be perceived and then through that perception one can understand what type of disorder is present.

Q: Since you have been trained in both allopathic and Ayurvedic systems of medicine, is this Ayurvedic concept of imbalance present somewhere in the traditional allopathic Western medical system?

A: Though the Western traditional medical system doesn't speak about imbalance, they do refer to disorders as psychosomatic disorders, or they may label something as a syndrome. Within the concept of disease they cannot pinpoint the disease, but call the set of symptoms a syndrome. Ayurveda says that these syndromes and sets of disorder are nothing but doshic changes. If vata is high a person gets constipation, gas, bloating, distention, and psychologically the person feels insecure and has insomnia. If such a patient visits a modern doctor, the doctor may tell them that they don't have a problem according to our definition of disease.

Q: The symptoms of imbalance are diagnosable by both systems of medicine, but it is the structure or the understanding of Ayurveda that collects the symptoms into a picture of imbalance.

A: Yes. Suppose a person has insomnia, lack of sleep. He goes to the doctor and they say, "Oh, he has insomnia that is not a disease," and the doctor prescribes a medicine to help the person sleep. Ayurveda would say, "Look, insomnia could be due to so many causes. What is the cause of this insomnia?" Is it a vata type of constipation causing insomnia, or too much work, worry, and stress? Or could it be due to a deadline at work and the person is under great pressure, which is a pitta imbalance? Then insomnia may be present from those factors. Ayurveda will not treat the symptom, but will treat the underlying definite cause of that symptom, and therefore, prevent the future recurrence of a disease. That is the difference between Ayurveda and modern medicine.

Q: What are the traditional Ayurvedic methods of assessment, such as pulse diagnosis or pulse assessment?

A: In Ayurvedic assessment of disease there are three basic methods: observation, palpation, and questioning. These are the basic methodologies used. They look at the person, look into the eyes, look at the tongue, observe the person's whole status, whether he is seriously or fatally ill, or there is a reasonably good prognosis. That observation opens new avenues of inquiry and investigation. Then, there is examination of pulse, which is a very important diagnostic tool in Ayurvedic medicine. The Ayurvedic physician feels the pulse to find out the person's dosha, prakruti (constitution), and vikruti (current state). There are other levels of the pulse that indicate the condition of the organs, tissues, and the subtypes of the doshas. All these subtleties can be observed and even the status of the person's pathogenesis can be determined through pulse examination.

Q: What treatment modalities are incorporated in Ayurvedic medicine?

A: Treatment is defined as the use of any method or means to establish the balance between the three doshas, the seven bodily tissues, the three bodily wastes, and the body/mind consciousness. This is called "chikitsa" and has two parts: shodana, which is detoxification when a person is strong enough to bear the strain of cleansing; and shamana, which is pacification or palliative measures when the patient is weak and cannot tolerate the stress of shodana.

There are five kinds of detoxification therapies, or shodana, used when the patient is strong enough to do them. They are purgation, vomiting, enema, medications administered by the nasal passages, and cleansing of the blood. Then there are seven types of shamana, or palliative measures. These involve kindling the gastric fire or one's digestive capacity; burning toxins with certain herbal combinations; detoxifying fasts such as a monodiet or juice fast, or observing and modifying water intake; specific types of exercise that bring balance such as yoga, sunbathing or moon-bathing; and, breathing techniques that restore balance to the doshas. Once detoxification is complete, rejuvenation (rasayana chikitsa) is called for. This helps maintain the patient's newly restored health and revitalizes him or her.

Q: Does removal of the cause fit into the classical Ayurvedic treatment modalities?

A: Yes. Ayurveda says nidana, or avoiding the cause, is a treatment. If a person has specific causes that aggravate vata, pitta, or kapha then we can avoid those causes. The body knows how to heal itself.

Q: We have a saying, "An ounce of prevention is worth a pound of cure." Is there some similar emphasis in Ayurveda on prevention and daily routine?

A: Yes. Prevention is better than cure. Prevention takes place through avoidance of cause, proper diet, lifestyle, and avoidance of certain situations where a person becomes aggravated and disturbed. That is true; prevention is much better than cure.

Q: What are some of the strengths of Ayurveda?

A: As we already discussed, Ayurveda heals by way of management. The most important strength of Ayurveda is the prakruti/vikruti paradigm. Ayurveda believes that every individual is a unique phenomenon. Every individual has a unique constitution. Therefore, Ayurveda tries to bring balance in the constitutional factors, or the three constitutional organizations of vata, pitta, and kapha. The present altered status of the dosha is called vikruti. Vikruti may not be necessarily a disease, but vikruti creates a potential for disease. One of the strengths of Ayurveda is to understand the present doshic status (vikruti) and what the original constitution was at the time of conception (prakruti) through Ayurvedic pulse diagnosis and other clinical assessments. The second important strength of Ayurveda is panchakarma, the cleansing program. This is a unique detoxification program based upon the prakruti/vikruti paradigm. The third important strength of Ayurveda is rasayana, or rejuvenation therapy. Probably the most important strength of Ayurveda is its knowledge of dinacharya, or daily routine. Daily routine can bring balance in any season and during most life changes. It helps you to maintain the balance of the three bodily organizations, vata, pitta, and kapha, according to the day, season, age, and specific disorders or disease. This knowledge is very powerful because Ayurveda believes proper diet is proper medicine and we must maintain balance between the internal ecology of the three doshas and one's external ecological and environmental changes. Another strength of Ayurveda is the art of longevity, living a long, happy, healthy, and holistic life established through a healthy daily routine.

Q: It seems true that a lot of responsibility is given to the patient or client to follow the guidelines. For people who want to do something themselves, daily routine is very good because it gives the individual positive steps to take.

A: Yes. And daily routine varies from person to person. At what time should one wake up and what should be done upon waking? One could start by brushing the teeth, scraping the tongue, drinking a glass of warm water, pranayama (breath techniques), meditation, yoga asanas, abhyanga (self-massage), bathing, and taking natural, herbal supplements. Making lifestyle changes empowers the individual. Ayurveda believes most disease begins due to wrong diet and wrong lifestyle and that we can avoid the major factors of disease just by following a proper daily routine.

Q: What evidence is there that Ayurveda works? If somebody said, "Prove to me that Ayurveda works," how would you answer that?

A: In Western herbal medicine they use milk thistle for the liver. In the same way, Ayurvedic herbal medicine uses kutki for liver detoxification. All ancient Ayurvedic herbal formulas and compounds like sitopaladi, mahasu-darshan, chandraprabha, and the compounds that are used in rheumatoid arthritis, are evidentially proven and time-proven medicines. They are given in the ancient texts as a specific medication and compound for specific conditions. And their effectiveness is empirically based. More recently, one of the Himalayan Ayurvedic herbal medicine companies has done research on a product called Liv-52. It contains 16 or 17 different herbs that are prepared in such a way that they detoxify the liver. They have done experiments where ethyl alcohol was injected into the liver of rats to induce alcoholic cirrhotic changes. They took biopsies from the rats and proved that there were microscopic cirrhotic changes. Then they gave the rats Liv-52 and within 100 days, a three-month period, the cirrhotic changes and the inflammatory changes healed. The company submitted this paper to medical doctors, and since then even medical doctors prescribe Liv-52. They think that Liv-52 is a modern drug! They don't really know that its origins are in the ancient texts of Ayurveda. I think Ayurveda is not only an evidentially and time-proven medicine; the Indian Research Council is doing research on several other Ayurvedic herbs like shatavari, brahmi, ash-waganda, and pippali.

Q: Is Ayurveda safe?

A: Ayurveda is absolutely safe. Ayurvedic herbal medicines use the whole plant. This is an important point because if we separate the chemically active ingredients of a particular plant, then it is no longer a natural Ayurvedic medicine; it becomes a chemical drug. And those drugs have side effects. Let's use guggulu as an example. Guggulu can be extremely toxic to the nervous system. If we separate the active ingredient, Factor A Gugguline and it is injected, it can create neurological tremors, fatigue, and sometimes a lack of coordination. That doesn't happen when we use guggulu as a whole. When we use Ayurvedic medicine according to Ayurvedic principles, it is quite safe. If we use modern concepts in Ayurvedic medicine and extract only one active ingredient, thinking that the rest of the plant or substance is "junk," that active ingredient alone can have hazardous side effects. Therefore, Ayurvedic herbal compounds are quite safe when we use whole herbal compounds and whole herbal remedies.

Q: **What about the use of preparations containing mercury, heavy metals, and bhasmas (chemical preparations known as ash) in Ayurveda? Can we assume that all the medicines we find available in today's market are properly prepared by competent pharmacies and that all of the ancient methods are being followed? Or is it more true that we have to be very careful these days because some of the ancient purification methods are lost and some of the companies take shortcuts.**

A: This is absolutely true because there are some companies that are commercialized and they don't follow the strict methods and means of preparing the herbal compounds. They fail to do this because they have a large number of orders and a great demand for their medicines. To supply that demand they skip some of the purification methods. For example, to make a gold bhasma is a time consuming procedure. If it is not done that way, the gold bhasma will be toxic to the system. If we use Ayurvedic medicine from an inauthentic source then yes, we may get hazardous, unwanted side effects. That is why it is very important to have proper medicine from an authentic Ayurvedic pharmaceutical company.

Q: **How can Ayurveda be integrated with conventional medicine?**

A: In the West, Ayurveda can be a great asset to modern medicine by advising the patient on proper diet and lifestyle using an individualistic approach, prakruti/vikruti balancing, and panchakarma (detoxification) and rasayana (rejuvenation) programs. Perhaps we would not use Ayurveda to handle acute emergencies, but more to deal with chronic problems like rheumatoid arthritis, sciatica, Parkinsonism, ascites, and hepatitis B and C. These are the areas where Ayurveda can be a great asset to modern medicine.

Q: **Are there any risks of interactions between Ayurvedic therapies and herbal products with conventional medicine? Should a physician be aware of certain interactions?**

A: I believe we can create integrated Ayurvedic clinics where modern medical doctors and Ayurvedic physicians work together; then Ayurvedic medicine can be a great asset to modern medicine. Suppose a person is receiving chemotherapy, which has pitta-provoking properties. People on chemotherapy lose their hair, get fevers, and their mucous lining becomes distorted. If we use Ayurvedic pitta-pacifying herbs, a cleansing program and diet, then the person can have good results without the side effects common to chemotherapy. Many modern medical drugs have side effects and there are even iatrogenic disorders or drug-induced diseases. Both can be effectively treated with Ayurvedic medicine. These are just a few examples of how Ayurveda could be a great asset to modern medicine when two professionals work together hand-in-hand.

There are always reactions between any modality and conventional medicine, even when it is an effective outcome. For this reason, the primary care provider should always be aware of the therapies the patient is undergoing. If the primary care provider does not communicate well with his patient and take a stand on knowing what the patient is taking, then there will be a problem.

Q: How is Ayurveda seen in Europe and in other parts of the world?

A: Ayurveda is seen the same as in the United States, even in Europe. In European countries when there is no further medical treatment, they look for homeopathic, naturopathic, or Ayurvedic assistance. They are hungry, like in the United States, to have an alternative measure for their modern medical treatments because every medical system has limitations and that's the beauty of it. Even Ayurveda has limitations. Homeopathy has limitations. Modern medicine has limitations. We can fill these gaps, these limitations with Ayurvedic medicine.

Q: Is Ayurveda still taught in conventional medical schools?

A: When I graduated, Pune University was teaching both modern and Ayurvedic medicine in tandem. That program ceased to exist. I think it is very important to have a parallel education in Ayurvedic and modern medicine so that the student will learn how Ayurveda can support their knowledge of tuberculosis in modern medicine, for example. In Ayurveda there are 20 different types of diabetes. Basically these 20 types are the complexities of diabetic syndrome. When a student learns in modern schools about diabetes, its etiology, pathology, symptomatology, and treatment, similarly they should learn Ayurvedic etiology, Ayurvedic pathology, Ayurvedic symptomatology, and treatment of diabetes. By studying these comparatively, they get new insights. I think there is no such school existing now.

Q: If somebody wants to become an Ayurvedic practitioner, how is that possible right now?

A: That is a very difficult question to answer. I think there are authentic Ayurvedic physicians, teachers, professors, and lecturers from whom people can learn Ayurveda. Modern medical science can be learned from a reputable medical school. Ideally, medical professionals could learn Ayurveda from institutions such as the Ayurvedic Institute. They can learn Ayurveda and bring with them the experience of their own background of allopathic, chiropractic, or even Chinese medicine. That may currently be the only realistic way to learn, incorporate, and practice Ayurvedic medicine. Regarding practice, it seems that a strong group could create its own lobby and its own authentic association that has a certification program, state examination program, and that teaches an authentic Ayurvedic curriculum. This is the future of Ayurveda.

Suggested Readings

Lad V. *Ayurveda: The Science of Self-Healing*. Twin Lakes, WI: Lotus Light Publications; 1984.

8

Homeopathy

Robert Leckridge, MBBCh, FFHoM

About the Author

Robert Leckridge graduated from Edinburgh University Medical School in 1978. With a strong ambition to be a family doctor since the age of 3, he began studying homeopathy in 1983 and found it easy to integrate into a busy National Health Service General Practice in Scotland. Time spent with patients taking a homeopathic perspective became so much more rewarding that he left General Practice in 1994 and took up a full-time position at Glasgow Homeopathic Hospital. He continues to work at Glasgow Homeopathic Hospital, both clinically and in teaching homeopathy to undergraduate and postgraduate healthcare professionals. In addition, he is the author of *Homeopathy in Primary Care* and was president of the UK Faculty of Homeopathy from 1999 to 2005.

Q: Tell me about how you got interested in homeopathic medicine.

A: I first expressed an interest in becoming a doctor when I was 3 years old. I can't remember a time when I had any other main goal. In fact, I didn't just want to be a doctor. I wanted to be a general practitioner (GP) or a "family doctor." My only model for a doctor was a series on Scottish TV when I was very young called "Dr. Finlay's Casebook." It was a kind of soap opera and Dr. Finlay was a GP in a small village only a few minutes from my home town of Stirling. I wanted to be like Dr. Finlay. Dr. Kildare was on our TV at that time too, but I didn't like him—that white-coated brashness put me off! So, after graduating from the University of Edinburgh in 1978, I completed GP Training over the following four years and then joined a small partnership of four GPs in a small Scottish village, Galston. I thought I had achieved my ambition—now I was Dr. Finlay!

In my second year in practice, I sat at the end of a morning clinic and asked myself, "What have I done for the patients I've seen this morning?" I knew I listened a lot, prescribed a lot of drugs (mainly anti-somethings like antihypertensives, anti-inflammatories, anti-depressants, etc.) and written some paperwork. What I didn't think I'd done was actually heal anyone. Where had that gotten lost?

If there was one reason why I wanted to be a doctor it was so I could help to heal people, so, as you can imagine, I was pretty unhappy to discover I wasn't doing that much. As luck, or God, or whatever, would have it, I received a letter in my mail that day advertising a course in homeopathy for GPs at the Glasgow Homeopathic Hospital. Well, I hadn't even heard the word "homeopathy" and had no idea what it was, but the advertisement attracted me. I can't remember the details, but it seemed like a good idea so I enrolled. After the first few days of the course, I started to try the homeopathic remedies I'd been taught and found to my surprise, delight, and amazement that they worked! The course taught us to use the remedies in situations where we didn't feel we had good orthodox alternatives, so I started using them to treat sports injuries, acute gastrointestinal infections, premenstrual syndrome, anticipatory anxiety, etc. I continued to use them in this limited way until I moved from Galston to join a friend in practice in Edinburgh. Within two weeks of starting in Edinburgh, I had patients coming to see me saying they heard I was a homeopath and they wanted a homeopathic treatment.

I had to admit I wasn't a homeopath and knew only a little homeopathy. This drove me to learn more and a few years later I qualified as a member of the Faculty of Homeopathy by passing their exacting national examination. Shortly after that, I began to work at the Glasgow Homeopathic Hospital in the Out-patient Department. I grew increasingly satisfied with the quality of my interactions with patients and the outcomes of the treatment and increasingly dissatisfied with the way GPs were forced to practice in the National Health Service. I resigned as a GP in 1994 and took up my present position at the Homeopathic Hospital. As if these changes were not radical enough, I also got deeply involved in teaching homeopathy and I now teach all round the world. I wrote a textbook of homeopathy, *Homeopathy in Primary Care,*[1] and I became the President of the Faculty of Homeopathy.

Q: What is homeopathy?

A: Homeopathy is a therapeutic approach that seeks to use naturally produced medicines to stimulate the body's own healing processes. It was invented by Dr. Samuel Hahnemann in the 18th century and it is based on two simple concepts: firstly, "like cures like" and, secondly, "use the minimum effective dose."

Q: Explain what "like cures like" means.

A: Hahnemann was translating the Pharmacopoea of the Scottish physician Cullen from English into German. He came across the description of the remedy "Peruvian Tree Bark" that was a treatment for swamp fever, or malaria. Cullen said this worked by being an astringent. Hahnemann wondered if this was true. To test it out, he took some of the medicine himself and much to his surprise discovered that he developed all the symptoms of someone who had swamp fever. This was the initial discovery: a drug which could cure a disease could also induce the same picture of the disease in a healthy person.

If you have ever had to look after an infant who has an acute fever, you'll be familiar with the picture of a child with high temperature: bright red cheeks, dilated pupils and dry mouth, maybe progressing to hallucinations and/or convulsions. This particular picture could be artificially produced in a toddler by poisoning them with Belladonna (Deadly Nightshade) which contains atropine-like chemicals. The homeopathic approach is to give a dose of Belladonna to this child and watch as the symptoms and the fever quickly subside. However, it really isn't a good idea to go around poisoning children, so Hahnemann thought, "I wonder how little of the medicine will cure the patient?" He prepared his medicines through a process of serial dilutions and successions. This resulted in drugs, or remedies as we call them, that were effective but so dilute they could not cause any poisoning.

Q: How is a homeopathic medicine prepared?

A: Homeopathic medicines are made from natural sources. About 70% of them are from plants, about 20% from minerals, and the rest from the animal kingdom. Many of the starting substances are highly toxic. The preparation involves diluting the starting material in alcohol, shaking it vigorously (traditionally by banging the test-tube repeatedly on a family bible), then taking a single drop of that dilution and adding it to the next container of alcohol. This process is repeated many times. There are two main scales of dilution commonly used: the "decimal" scale (represented by an "X" or "D" on the label) where each stage of preparation is 1:9, meaning one drop of the medicine to 9 drops of diluent; and the "centesimal" scale (represented by a "c" on the label) where each stage of preparation is 1:99. This is repeated many times, so a remedy described as "30c" has undergone 30 stages of dilution and succession. You'll have worked out that this is equivalent to a dilution of 100 to the power of 30 which is way beyond Avogadro's number so it is highly unlikely that there are any molecules of the starting material left in the "30c" remedy.

Q: If there are not any molecules present in the remedy, can it actually work?

A: It's a mystery! Clearly, it isn't a pharmacological effect. It isn't a molecular effect. There has been a lot of interesting work on ultra-high dilutions that indicates the information imparted by the substance to the diluent remains present even once the substance has gone. People call this "the memory of water." This seems like a major challenge to orthodox thinking, but I don't think it is such a huge challenge really. We are aware that many things can impact us physically and emotionally without conveying information on molecules, such as words, images, and music. We are influenced by information and signals all the time and much of this information is not carried on molecules. However, the ultra-high dilution research is looking interesting and I wouldn't be surprised to see a mechanism of action published in my lifetime.

Q: What evidence is there that homeopathy works, or that it is more than just a placebo?

A: These are two different questions, but I understand that they are related. We could have a big debate here about what constitutes evidence, but let me simply focus on the kind of evidence that most physicians accept, randomized clinical trials. There have been a couple of major meta-analyses of the published trials.[2,3] Both have shown that homeopathic treatments have an effect and both have shown that the evidence is weakly in favor of showing an effect that is greater than placebo. Dr. Robert Mathie[4] published an interesting analysis of the research trials recently and has found 50 papers which show a significant benefit of homeopathy in at least one clinical outcome measure and "the weight of evidence currently favors a positive treatment effect in eight [conditions]: childhood diarrhea, fibrositis, hayfever, influenza, pain, side-effects of radio- and chemo-therapy, sprains and upper respiratory tract infection."

However, let me just refer to another area of study, outcomes research. There have been a number of outcomes studies published by the Homeopathic Hospitals in the United Kingdom. What they all show is that the people treated at these hospitals have usually already tried the best orthodox treatments but still have their suffering. In approximately 70% of these people treated homeopathically, they claim a reduction of their symptoms and an increase in their well-being sufficient to make a significant difference in their daily lives. This is certainly my daily experience. This approach relieves suffering in patients who have not found relief in the best evidence-based treatments.

Q: What's involved in a homeopathic consultation?

A: A homeopathic consultation for a new patient will take at least an hour. It is a comprehensive medical history that pays great attention to enabling the patient to tell the story of his or her own experience in his or her own words. Much of the history covers the same ground as a good traditional medical history. We start with the presenting complaint. My first question to a patient is usually, "I've received a referral letter from your doctor, but that really is just an introduction. I wonder if you could just tell me your own story in your own words?" This is quite an unusual start to a consultation and some patients are initially a bit taken aback by it, but soon they get into their story. I want to know everything they can tell me about their illness experience. What are their symptoms? What exactly do these symptoms feel like? Where do the symptoms occur? What influences the symptoms? When did they start? Then we move on to cover the past medical history, the family history, social history, their allergies, women's menstrual patterns. Following that, I check to see if there are any other problems they haven't mentioned by doing a systematic review. All of this is just a good straightforward medical history. I'll move on to ask the patient to describe some things about themselves that doctors don't usually inquire about. In homeopathy we call these the "generals," or a way to check the person's responses to environmental influences. I ask if they are affected by any particular weather, by heat or cold. I ask about perspiration, about their daily cycles of energy, about sleep and dreams, about appetite and their relationship to food-stuffs—cravings, aversions, foods that upset. I ask about thirst and how they quench it. The final section of the history gives me an idea of their character, emotional life, and cognitive function. This final section is quite like a mental state inquiry used in psychiatry.

Q: Why do you ask all this detail?

A: I need to know what makes this person unique. How do they uniquely experience their illness and how do they cope with it. I'm looking for the stand-out symptoms, the important ones to the patient and the ones that individualize the story. Take 100 patients with asthma. They'll all have certain common symptoms that lead to the diagnosis of asthma. But if these 100 patients all had asthma for a number of years, they will all have developed different patterns of experience and different ways of coping. It's these latter features that show their differences. Once I've identified the unique patterns, I try to match them to the patterns of illness described in the homeopathic literature. There are about 3000 remedies to choose from, and each one has a detailed description of the patterns they can match.

Q: Where does this information come from?

A: It comes from three sources:

- Provings—This was a method invented by Hahnemann. It consists of giving a remedy to a group of healthy volunteers and recording their experience.
- Toxicology of the starting substances—The example I gave earlier of Belladonna gives you an idea of how this works.
- Evidence of 200 years of clinical practice—When a patient responded well to a homeopathic remedy, the homeopaths recorded the patterns which the patients had exhibited.

Q: Having found the match, what do you do next?

A: I prescribe a single dose of the remedy that best matches the case. Then I ask the patient to return in about a month and tell me what, if any, kind of reaction they get to that remedy.

Q: Why only one dose?

A: Well, it's not a drug. It's not working by suppressing anything, like a painkiller. Instead it is a stimulus to the body's healing system. It's like giving it a prod! Sometimes I use the analogy of immunization to explain it to my patients. I say, "If I wanted to immunize you against polio today, I'd put three polio drops on your tongue and send you home." I wouldn't say, "Here's a litre of polio. Take a tablespoonful a day for the rest of your life." They usually laugh and understand exactly what I'm saying. I say, "Homeopathy is a bit like that. I'm just giving something for your healing system to respond to. I'm not trying to damp something down."

Q: How can homeopathy be incorporated in conventional medicine?

A: The outcomes research hints at how homeopathy can be incorporated into conventional medicine. Broadly, I'd highlight four ways in which it can be incorporated.

1. In the treatment of conditions for which there are no effective orthodox interventions.

   Infant colic is a good example. There really aren't any safe, effective drugs for this condition, which causes great distress to infants and parents alike. However, homeopathic remedies like colocynth can relieve the pain in many of these babies within minutes.

2. In situations where we have effective treatments, but the side-effects are unacceptable.

   An example of this would be the use of non-steroidal anti-inflammatories in the treatment of patients with arthritis. Thousands of people are admitted to hospitals every year with gastrointestinal bleeding caused by these drugs. Many of these patients could have their pain relieved with harmless homeopathic medicines instead.

3. In situations where effective treatments are contra-indicated.

   For example, in treating pregnancy sickness where anti-nausea drugs are not safe to use.

4. To reduce the long-term need for drugs to control chronic conditions.

   Conditions like epilepsy and psoriasis are likely to require life-long medication. Homeopathic medicines can reduce the severity and frequency of flare-ups and, therefore, reduce the need for such large quantities of drugs.

Q: **Are there any risks of interactions between homeopathic remedies and conventional medicines?**

A: No. Remedies, I often say to my patients, do nothing. (I tend to pause there for dramatic effect!) All they do is stimulate the body's own healing processes. If you experience improvement it is because your healing system is doing its job. The remedies are not drugs. We have already established that they don't act pharmacologically. They will not interfere with conventional drugs. Indeed, the two approaches can work well hand-in-hand. As drugs dampen down distressing or even life-threatening symptoms, the remedy can stimulate the natural repair and recovery. There is a belief that powerful drugs will inhibit the effect of remedies. This is true because some powerful drugs (e.g., steroids and chemotherapy) do impede the body's healing responses, and by so doing, will interfere with the action of a remedy. I think this issue is rather overplayed, however, as we have many patients in Glasgow Homeo-pathic Hospital who are admitted on powerful drugs that can't be stopped and we still see results from the homeopathic treatments.

Q: **Are remedies safe?**

A: Yes, they are non-toxic. As Professor Ernst of Exeter University, who has studied homeopathy, has said, "Homeopathic remedies seem to be safe. It's the homeopaths who are not always safe." He surveyed the world literature for evidence of reports of harm from the use of homeopathy and that was his conclusion.

Q: **Is homeopathic medicine taught in conventional medical schools?**

A: Homeopathic medicine is usually taught post-graduation. The Faculty of Homeopathy in the United Kingdom, for example, only trains statutorily reg-istered healthcare professionals. This picks up Professor Ernst's point about the safety of practitioners. In many countries people practice homeopathy without any official registration as a healthcare professional. This tends to mean that they have not had the benefit of a full training such as that received by doctors, nurses, dentists, and so on. There are many skills needed to prac-tice well and safely as a healthcare professional and learning the homeopathic method is only a part of that. In recent years, many universities have begun to include familiarization courses in a number of complementary therapies.

Q: How is homeopathic medicine seen in Europe and other parts of the world?

A: The laws governing the practice of medicine are different throughout the world. That's one of the problems that homeopathic medicine faces. If you live in a country where you can advertise yourself as a homeopath without any training and without any regulation, then what kind of message does that send out about homeopathy? If it is an effective and a significant treatment, then it deserves to be taken seriously and not practiced as a hobby. Conventional biomedical thinking sticks on the issue of the high dilutions and the evidence-based medicine bandwagon and has marginalized the wealth of experience of patients and of doctors who have used homeopathy. Both patients and healthcare professionals are increasingly dissatisfied with the current reductionist thinking. I have worked through the Faculty of Homeopathy to respond to requests for the development of homeopathic training courses in several countries in recent years and we are currently actively providing training in the United Kingdom, Portugal, Russia, Japan, South Africa, and India. People are voting with their feet and beating a path to the homeopathic training programs and the homeopathic clinics.

Q: Are there conditions that conventional medicine cannot help and homeopathy can?

A: It's really all about a difference in approach. Conventional medicine is terrific at acute medicine. Our technologies have mainly been directed at saving lives. This is good, because if you don't save a life, you have no patient to treat! However, it is no secret that conventional medicine really struggles to treat chronic diseases. I think this is where a therapy like homeopathy excels. If the body's healing system is working well, the chronic illnesses cause less trouble. The patient copes better and has a better experience of health.

Q: There are many side effects to conventional treatments, specifically pharmacological complications of treatment of disease. How can a perspective of homeopathy help the patient achieve optimal health in situations where conventional medications or treatments have more negative side effects?

A: Homeopathy can minimize the need for drugs, reduce the doses required, and, thereby, reduce the chances of experiencing side effects by decreasing the number of acute attacks within a chronic disease, reducing symptoms experienced on a daily basis, and stimulating the healing system.

Q: Who can use homeopathic treatments safely, and who should be careful when using homeopathic treatments?

A: Homeopathic remedies are completely safe in all kinds of situations. They can be used safely in newborn infants, in elderly patients with multiple pathologies, and in patients who have impaired renal or hepatic function.

Q: How can I become a homeopathic practitioner?

A: First, I'd ask what kind of healthcare professional you are. Are you a doctor, a veterinarian, a nurse, a dentist . . . ? Whatever your professional discipline, you can learn homeopathy and integrate it into your practice.

What our students tell us is that learning the homeopathic method affects their daily practice. They begin to enjoy their job again and as their patients' satisfaction increases, so does their professional satisfaction. If you want to learn homeopathy as a professional skill I would suggest you contact your national professional homeopathic medical organization and ask about available courses.

Suggested Readings

National Center for Homeopathy. Available at: http://www.homeopathic.org

North American Society of Homeopaths (NASH) available at: http://www.homeopathy.org

Faculty of Homeopathy (UK). Available at: www.trusthomeopathy.org/faculty

American Institute of Homeopathy (USA). Available at: www.homeopathyusa.org

The British Homeopathic Association. Available at: www.trusthomeopathy.org

The Glasgow Homeopathic Hospital. Available at: www.hom-inform.org

Enable Learning. Available at: www.enablelearning.net

References

1. Leckridge R. *Homeopathy in Primary Care*. Edinburgh, London: Churchill Livingston; 1997.

2. Kleijnen J, Knipschild P, Ter Riet G. (1991). Clinical trials of homeopathy. *British Med J*. 1991;302(6TT2):316–323.

3. Linde K, Clausius N, Ramirez G, Melchart D, et al. Are the clinical effects of homoeopathy placebo effects? A meta-analysis of placebo-controlled trials. *Lancet*. 1997;350(9081):834–843.

4. Mathie R. The research evidence base for homeopathy; a fresh assessment of the literature. *Homeopathy*. 2003;92(2):84–91.

9

Naturopathic Medicine

Michael Traub, ND, DHANP, CCH

About the Author

Michael Traub was the first naturopathic physician in contemporary times to be appointed to a hospital staff at North Hawaii Community Hospital (NHCH). Dr. Traub served as president of the American Association of Naturopathic Physicians (AANP) from 2001 to 2003 and has held numerous other leadership positions within the naturopathic profession throughout his career, from chairman of the Hawaii Board of Naturopathic Examiners to president of the Homeopathic Academy of Naturopathic Physicians and president of the North American Board of Naturopathic Examiners. Since 1986, Dr. Traub has been director of an integrated healthcare center (Lokahi Health Center) in Kailua Kona, Hawaii, and he also has a part-time practice in Marin County, California. Information available at **www.balancerestored.com**.

Q: Tell me about how you got interested in naturopathic medicine.

A: I wanted to be a doctor for as long as I could remember. My father was a dermatologist, my mother a nurse. While pre-med in college, I met a medical student who, when he graduated as valedictorian, said the following at the commencement ceremony: "I cannot in good conscience practice medicine. I have been stripped of my humanity and trained to be a technician." When I heard this, it opened my awareness that perhaps there was another way to become a doctor. When I discovered the profession of naturopathic medicine, I knew it was the right blend of modern science and holistic medicine that I wanted to practice.

Q: What is naturopathy?

A: Naturopathy blends centuries-old natural, non-toxic therapies with current advances in medicine, covering all aspects of health from prenatal to geriatric care. Naturopathic medicine:

- Concentrates on whole-person wellness. The treatment is tailored to the patient and emphasizes prevention and self-care.
- Attempts to find the underlying cause of the patient's condition rather than focusing solely on symptomatic treatment.
- Is defined primarily by its fundamental principles
  - First do no harm
  - The healing power of nature
  - Treat the cause
  - Treat the whole person
  - Doctor as teacher
  - Prevention

- Methods and modalities are selected and applied based upon these principles in relationship to the individual needs of each patient. Diagnostic and therapeutic methods are selected from various sources and systems and continue to evolve with the progress of knowledge.
- Includes the following diagnostic and therapeutic modalities: all methods of clinical and laboratory diagnosis including diagnostic imaging; nutritional, botanical, and homeopathic medicine; acupuncture and Chinese medicine; naturopathic physical medicine including physiotherapy, hydrotherapy, manipulation, and therapeutic exercise; psychotherapy and counseling; minor surgery; and natural childbirth.

Q: Explain how naturopathic medicine works.

A: Naturopathic medicine supports and promotes the body's natural healing process leading to the highest state of wellness. By addressing the causes of disease and individualizing treatment that integrates the healing powers of body, mind and spirit, health can be restored, optimized, and maintained.

Q: Is naturopathic medicine safe?

A: Yes. The safety record in states with regulatory boards is excellent. Naturo-pathic physicians can purchase malpractice insurance at extremely low rates. As indicated by such rates, the chance of being injured through mal-practice is low. Naturopathic physicians are experts in the safe use of natu-ral therapies.

Q: What evidence is there that naturopathic medicine works?

A: Naturopathic medicine has its own unique body of knowledge, evolved and refined for centuries. It also incorporates scientific advances from medical disciplines throughout the world. Many of the individual therapies of naturopathic medical practice have been scientifically validated, especially in the areas of clinical nutrition, botanical medicine, homeopathy, acupunc-ture, and manipulation. The trend is that those naturopathic methods which are tested in well-designed studies are validated. Research is presently being conducted on the effectiveness of the whole system of natur-opathy when it is applied to patients with certain conditions.

Q: How can naturopathy be blended with conventional medicine?

A: Naturopathic medicine shares a foundation of diagnostic methods with conventional medicine. Although treatment approaches may differ, they are not mutually exclusive. Many patients are under the care of both a conven-tional physician and a naturopathic physician, utilizing the strengths and avoiding the shortcomings of each approach. In an ideal world, patients would have the benefit of the best of both systems. Naturopathy has effec-tive treatment for many problems that conventional medicine fails to cure, such as asthma, arthritis, migraine, diabetes, and hypertension. Recently, conventional medicine has incorporated some naturopathic wisdom in the areas of nutrition, diet, exercise therapy, and mind-body correlations.

Q: Are there any risks of interactions between natural medicines and conven-tional medicines?

A: Yes. Many patients are blending the use of natural medicines and conven-tional medicine. The knowledge base about herb, nutrient, and drug interac-tions is rapidly expanding. Naturopathic physicians are experts in the safe use of natural medicines and prescription drugs. In my article "Reconsider-ing Supplemental Pharmaceutical Interactions," I discussed some examples of supplement-pharmaceutical interactions.[1]

Q: Is naturopathic medicine taught in conventional medical schools?

A: No. Conventional medical schools may offer introductory courses on the modalities of naturopathic medicine such as clinical nutrition, botanical medicine, and homeopathy, and may provide an overview of naturopathy.

But, naturopathy is not currently part of the core curriculum of any conventional medical school in North America.

Q: Has conventional medicine adopted methods from the naturopathic body of knowledge?

A: Yes. The dangers of harmful fats, excess carbohydrates, and inadequate fiber are now accepted in conventional medicine. The benefits of whole foods, medicinal plants, exercise, and the influence of mental and emotional attitudes on health are all part of the naturopathic body of knowledge. As mentioned above, some of this knowledge has been incorporated into conventional medicine in the last few years.

Q: How is naturopathic medicine seen in Europe and other parts of the world?

A: Although complementary and alternative medicine is more accepted in Europe and other parts of the world, the profession of naturopathic medicine is not as well-developed as it is in North America. Other countries are looking to the Unites States and Canada to model their naturopathic medical programs and professions. While serving as president of the American Association of Naturopathic Physicians, I was a featured speaker at the first International Congress of Naturopathy held in Spain in 2003.

Q: How is naturopathic medicine different from conventional medicine?

A: The main difference is in philosophical approach. Naturopathic physicians treat patients by restoring overall health rather than suppressing a few key symptoms. Naturopathic physicians are more concerned with finding the underlying cause of a condition and applying treatments that work in alliance with the natural healing mechanisms of the body rather than against them. Naturopathic treatments result less frequently in adverse side effects or in the chronic conditions that inevitably arise when the cause of disease is left untreated. Naturopathic physicians typically spend more time with patients, taking a more comprehensive approach and spending time with education and answering questions.

Q: What is the difference between naturopathy and homeopathy?

A: Naturopathy encompasses the entire spectrum of natural medicine, of which homeopathy is just one part. Homeopathy is a system which utilizes extremely small doses of natural substances to stimulate the body's own ability to heal, and thus is based on many of the same principles as naturopathy—treating the cause, treating the whole person, doing no harm, and utilizing the healing power of nature. Homeopathy is part of the foundation of naturopathic medicine, yet it may be taught and practiced just by itself and by healthcare providers who are not naturopathic physicians.

Q: Are there conditions that conventional medicine cannot help but naturopathy can?

A: Yes. Naturopathy outshines conventional medicine in conditions such as chronic fatigue syndrome, fibromyalgia, recurrent ear infections, and acute viral infections such as the flu and the common cold.

Q: Who can use naturopathic treatments safely?

A: Pregnant women, newborns, all phases of life up to geriatric care, and terminally ill persons can benefit safely from naturopathic medicine.

Q: How can I become a naturopathic physician?

A: Complete a college degree and meet the requirements for admission to one of the five accredited naturopathic medical schools in North America (**Table 9.1**).

Applicants are considered on the basis of academic performance, maturity, and demonstrated humanitarian qualities. Work and volunteer experience in health care coupled with an awareness of the field of natural medicine is desired. Students attend a four-year graduate-level naturopathic medical program and are educated in the same basic sciences as in conventional medical school. Upon completion of the graduation requirements, the student is awarded a Doctor of Naturopathic Medicine degree (ND). Graduates sit for professional board exams to become licensed as general practice naturopathic doctors within licensed states or as individual jurisdictions allow.

Q: What does the education of a naturopathic physician entail?

A: The first two years of naturopathic medical school consist of basic medical sciences such as anatomy, physiology, biochemistry, physical and clinical diagnosis, laboratory diagnosis, etc. The second two years emphasize the

Table 9.1 Accredited Naturopathic Medical Schools in North America

Member Institutions of the American Association of Naturopathic Medical Colleges	
Bastyr University	Kenmore, WA
Canadian College of Naturopathic Medicine	Toronto, Ontario, Canada
National College of Naturopathic Medicine	Portland, OR
Southwest College of Naturopathic Medicine	Tempe, AZ
University of Bridgeport College of Naturopathic Medicine	Bridgeport, CT
Candidate Program: Boucher Institute of Naturopathic Medicine	New Westminster, BC, Canada

application of naturopathic therapies such as clinical nutrition, botanical medicine, homeopathy, physical medicine, and lifestyle counseling to the entire range of human diseases in courses on gynecology, obstetrics, pediatrics, neurology, endocrinology, cardiology, pulmonology, urology, dermatology, and immunology. Clinical training and therapeutic education are integrated throughout the final academic years. Naturopathic philosophy is integrated throughout the curriculum. As all doctors in practice know, their education continues throughout their career.

Q: Is naturopathic medicine new?

A: It formed as a distinct American medical profession in 1902. In the 100 years of its existence, naturopathy has evolved into a sophisticated approach to natural health care while retaining the principles and some of the traditional approaches upon which it was founded. It is constantly evolving and adapting to the ever-growing body of medical knowledge, both conventional and naturopathic.

Q: In what ways are naturopathic and conventional physicians alike?

A: The academic training in medical sciences of naturopathic and conventional physicians is similar. Both study modern physical, clinical, and laboratory diagnosis. Both can diagnose a disease and predict its course. Naturopathic physicians also perform minor surgery and prescribe some drugs. Both naturopathic and conventional physicians refer patients to other healthcare practitioners when appropriate.

Q: Are naturopathic physicians opposed to drugs and major surgery?

A: No. Naturopathic physicians are not opposed to invasive or suppressive measures when these methods are necessary. They make referrals for such treatment when appropriate. Naturopathic medicine has both safer and less expensive alternatives to many kinds of non-emergency surgery.

Q: Where are naturopathic physicians licensed?

A: Alaska, Arizona, California, Connecticut, Hawaii, Idaho, Kansas, Maine, Montana, New Hampshire, Oregon, Utah, Vermont, Washington, Washington DC, Puerto Rico, and the Virgin Islands all license naturopathic physicians. Florida still has NDs practicing, but has not issued any new licenses in many years. In Canada, NDs are licensed in Ontario, British Columbia, Manitoba, and Saskatchewan. However, doctors of naturopathic medicine practice in most states and provinces, sometimes under other medical licenses and sometimes with a scope of practice substantially less than their training. There are 24 state naturopathic medical associations in the Unites States and Naturopathic licensure campaigns are underway in several states and provinces.

Q: Are there other kinds of NDs in the Unites States?

A: Because naturopathic medicine is not regulated in all 50 states, some individuals who call themselves naturopaths do not meet the historical standards of the profession. Such individuals sometimes have degrees or diplomas from correspondence schools, weekend seminar programs without supervised clinical training, extremely abbreviated courses, "certifying" agencies that confer naturopathic credentials based on other kinds of health education, "home study" schools without state authority to grant degrees, or schools without naturopathic programs or faculty. None of these programs qualify a candidate to sit for licensing board exams or to receive licensure in any state. In some states, individuals call themselves "naturopaths" simply by paying a fee for a business license requiring no evidence of education at all. There are a growing number of correspondence schools claiming to offer educational programs leading to the ND degree. Buyer beware is the rule here, both for those seeking a healthcare provider and for those thinking about a career. Consumers should know what they are getting when they seek the services of a naturopathic physician. Only licensure can guarantee the training and safety to which consumers are entitled.

Q: Is naturopathic medicine covered by insurance?

A: Yes, many insurance carriers cover naturopathic medicine in the Unites States and Canada. State legislatures in Connecticut, Washington, Montana, and Alaska have mandated insurance reimbursement for medically necessary and appropriate naturopathic medical services. However, all insurance companies vary regarding their coverage; therefore, it is very important for people to check their individual insurance policies to verify exactly what their policy covers.

Q: Is naturopathic medicine cost effective?

A: Yes, because naturopathic physicians have alternatives to some expensive high-tech procedures, and because their preventative approach reduces the incidence of high-cost chronic conditions, naturopathic practice reduces both immediate and long-term healthcare costs.

Suggested Readings

American Association of Naturopathic Physicians. Available at: http://naturopathic.org

American Association of Naturopathic Medical Colleges. Available at: http://www.aanmc.org/about.shtml

Pizzorno J, Murray M. *Textbook of Natural Medicine*. 3rd ed. New York, NY: Churchill Livingstone; 2005.

References

1. Traub, M. Reconsidering supplement-pharmaceutical interactions. *Holistic Primary Care*. 2002;3(3). Available at: http://holisticprimarycare.net/appl/ category23.jsp

10

Biofeedback

G. Frank Lawlis, PhD

About the Author

G. Frank Lawlis has focused upon clinical and research methods of the mind-body relationship since 1968 when he received his PhD in Counseling Psychology with an emphasis in medical psychology and rehabilitation. He has been awarded the Diplomate (ABPP) in both Counseling Psychology and Clinical Psychology. He also received the status of Fellow from the American Psychological Association for his scientific contributions to the field of clinical psychology and behavioral medicine, and he has been honored with numerous other awards for his pioneering research in this field. Lawlis has authored and co-authored six books: *Imagery and Disease, Bridges of the Bodymind, Transpersonal Medicine, Caregivers Guide to the Cure: The Hero's Journey with Cancer, Complementary and Alternative Medicine Management: Forms and Guidelines,* and *Mosby's Complementary and Alternative Medicine: A Research-Based Approach.* In addition, he has written more than 100 articles and chapters in various publications.

Q: What got you interested in biofeedback as a type of complementary and alternative medicine?

A: In 1967, when I was doing my residency in clinical psychology at New York University, I heard lecturer Neal Miller. He was explaining his research with his rats and we had a lengthy discussion afterwards about the implications for human problems. It was great and I started my pilgrimage into learning about what physiological measures could be measured and had relevance to real world problems.

The first thing I remember was getting a fish catch monitor, a mechanism that made a buzz when the line was drawn and signifying a weight at the end, presumably a fish. I tied the monitor to lines crossing the back of a scoliosis patient to give him feedback on straightening his back. It looked like a web. It was moderately successful and the patient was enthusiastic, but the technology was weak.

Q: Why do you believe in biofeedback?

A: I believe in biofeedback because the patients believe in it. They see results and come to believe in themselves, in their imagery and creativity, and in their abilities to heal themselves. The thing I enjoy most is that it becomes more of a coaching relationship that we are going to win rather than a "what-is-wrong-with-me" relationship. It is an empirical approach in which we can see how we are doing.

Q: Does biofeedback really work?

A: Biofeedback is a technology that can be used with many therapies. It is really a validity check on what the goals are of a therapy. If you are working on balance and you use scales as your feedback, you know if the therapy is working. If you are working with imagery in increasing the blood flow to your bones so they will mend faster or to fend off a migraine headache by using a temperature device, then you gain validity in the approach you are using.

Q: How does it work?

A: Biofeedback works like a mirror to your physiology. For example, if you want to learn to wiggle your ears, you look into the mirror and monitor what you have to do to get them moving. If you want the blood to flow at a higher rate in your hand, you monitor a temperature device that correlates with blood flow. If you want to learn to relax your muscles, you monitor an electromyogram monitor (EMG) and find ways, such as breathing, imagery, posturing, or other ways to achieve those goals. The question of "How does it work?" is answered best by "How well do you learn?"

Q: What are the physical mechanisms of healing?

A: The healing mechanisms are based on the etiologies of the problems. For example, most of the problems seen in a biofeedback lab come from chronic stress. Chronic stress can affect your immune system, your pain tolerance, and your healing process. By relieving the stress component, the body is allowed to mend itself naturally. Biofeedback can also enhance the healing process by increasing blood flow to an area, perhaps increasing white blood efficiency as well. And EMG biofeedback can help develop proper muscle balance in rehabilitation.

Q: What is the relationship between mind and body?

A: As Candace Pert and other pioneers have shown, the head bone is connected to the toe bone and all parts between. Stress has been shown to affect virtually every system we have, even to how we grow hair. Sports psychology research has shown that performance is maximized with appropriate mind states. No one can argue with relationship; however, it is still a mystery that many medical specialties still do not account for this issue.

Q: Is this mind over matter?

A: This is not mind over matter because a person is not doing something unnatural. The process is to ensure natural healing through improved skills of the person. It is interesting that many people have never been taught self-healing skills, possibly because we are given pills and rely on the surgeon so much.

Q: Is this part of a religious movement?

A: Biofeedback received the connotation of being part of Transcendental Meditation when early researchers, such as Elmer Green, were investigating the brain states of meditators. Actually the instrumentation was biofeedback equipment, but the individuals were not doing feedback. But there are people who still relate the two fields.

Q: Is this like hypnosis?

A: Maybe the two are linked because hypnosis and biofeedback both focus a lot on relaxation strategies. Few hypnotherapists use the instrumentation; however, I have found it extremely useful to use some monitoring on the part of the therapist to determine what suggestions are being effective for the patients to relax. For example, a number of hypnotherapists use scripts that have been successful in the past, such as suggesting listening to beach sounds as a helpful imagery for relaxation. But when I hooked up a number of patients to a galvanic skin conduction machine that records immediate emotional sensitivity, a number of these patients did not respond to these images. When asked about their responses, these individuals also reported no conscious affect of the imagery. In other words, no therapist can know exactly how a person is responding to suggestions and it is helpful to have an indication.

Q: Does it hurt? Do you get shocked?

A: The question of electric shock often arises when people see the equipment and have electrical patches placed on them. There is no danger of electrical shock because there is no electrical current going to them. Moreover, the equipment is more like a voltage meter that measures electrical energy coming from the patient that is correlated to the electrical energy the body gives off due to muscle tension or brain wave activity.

Q: Is it good only for one or two problems or does it cure everything?

A: Biofeedback is not a cure-all. As indicated above, most of the benefits of biofeedback relate to stress management skills and training of compromised neuromuscular systems. A short list of the most successful categories of problems treated by biofeedback approaches is as follows:
- Headaches (tension and migraine)
- Low back pain
- Temporomandibula jaw pain
- Neuromuscular dysfunction and paralysis
- Essential hypertension
- Other cardiovascular problems, such as arrhythmias
- Immune function related to stress reduction
- Arthritis treatment
- Disorders of the digestive system
- Incontinence
- Anxiety and panic disorders
- Attention Deficit Disorder (ADD)
- Raynard's Disease
- Epilepsy
- Stress management
- Premenstrual syndrome
- Sleep problems

Q: Is it contraindicated for some people or problems?

A: Biofeedback treatment, especially for stress, is contraindicated for depressed patients and for some people with histories with Epilepsy seizures as well as under supervision with diabetes. The reasons are obvious. For depressed people who are already low in energy, the lowering of their energies for the sake of stress management makes them anxious. People with Epilepsy histories often are stimulated for further seizures by lowering their brain wave patterns to those known to induce these activities; however, there are specific biofeedback programs that can help people minimize seizures through excitement, not reduction of brain wave activity. I feel that people with diabetes should be carefully monitored because insulin production and efficiency is so related to stress of the individual. If a person with high insulin needs gets relaxed, the internal insulin can flood the system and may cause some insulin shock symptoms. These are not serious if recognized and responded to promptly.

Q: **Does biofeedback work with everybody?**

A: Biofeedback does not work for everybody. In fact, I would probably guess that it would not work for the majority of the country because in order to be successful in healing yourself, you have to be motivated to take charge of your life and learn the skills necessary to change your life. My impression is that people who go into their doctors' office do not want to change their lives in order to be healed. Look at the people who smoke in the face of overwhelming evidence that smoking can be a major factor in illness. Look at the overweight people who refuse to change their diets even though obesity is a major factor in illness. The majority of our citizens will not exercise at the minimum level even though exercise is the healthiest thing anyone could do for health and it is free.

In biofeedback, I ask people to change their lives and if they do, they learn the lessons of self-healing. In light of how many people who will not change their life, how can anyone expect any type of self-help to work? Biofeedback requires self-awareness, the motivation to understand oneself, and to do what is necessary.

Q: **Do biofeedback treatments last?**

A: The interesting fact of biofeedback is that it is based on a learning model and once a pattern of healing is learned, it often becomes unconscious. For example, the patient with hypertension due to chronic stress learns to relax and lower his blood pressure. After months of practicing his approach, it becomes reflexive and lasting.

Q: **How many people use biofeedback?**

A: When I contacted the Association for Applied Psychophysiology and Biofeedback about membership, they indicated that they have over 2000 practicing members; however, biofeedback has been around for over 30 years as a profession. The answer would be in the millions, but I could only guess as to a specific number.

Q: **What type of research has been done in biofeedback?**

A: It is my opinion that biofeedback has been researched more than any other treatment modality. It has a journal dedicated to clinical research (*Journal of Applied Psychophysiology and Biofeedback*), and the applications continue to be researched for new approaches for new problems. I would recommend the chapter on biofeedback research in the *Mosby Textbook for Complementary and Alternative Medicine* for a summary of substantiated research.[1]

Q: How much does biofeedback cost?

A: The question of cost is based on who administers the treatment rather than what treatments are administered. If a clinical psychologist administers biofeedback, the fee will be based on clinical psychology in that area. If a physical therapist administers the treatment, the fees for physical therapists apply. The basis for this arrangement comes from the notion that broader scope of treatments are integrated with higher level expertise.

Q: Does insurance reimburse you for treatment?

A: It depends on the insurance coverage as to whether an insurance company covers the fees. Biofeedback services often come under the category of mental health or physical therapy. Most practitioners do not have to have a physician's prescription for administering biofeedback. It is often used as an integrated treatment under the supervision of a physician, therefore, insurance companies usually require a prescription for payment.

Q: Are there any consequences to your health?

A: Biofeedback has no known negative side-effects since the patient is under complete control of the learning process. Unlike medications that affect the whole body without control once the person has digested them, biofeedback is a form of learning physiological control. By controlling your own process of learning, you can control side-effects.

Q: How do you know if it is working and not a result of something else?

A: The main point of knowing whether it is working is biofeedback. If it is working, it is validated instantly. For example, if you are trying to relax your lumbar muscles in order to relieve your back pain, and you are trying to accomplish this goal by focusing on your breathing patterns, you will know by the feedback of the machines that you are accomplishing your goals. If not, you try something else until you can see and hear (via audio sounds) that you are successful.

Q: What will my doctor think of this?

A: Due to the research and demonstrations, most doctors have heard of biofeedback and know that it is not harmful to anything they are providing. They may not be enthusiastic because they have not experienced it, but I have never heard of anyone bashing it. In fact, 75% of the time doctors have recommended biofeedback if the patient asks about it and 25% will recommend it if they know someone who can offer reliable services in the area.

Q: Do I need to approve biofeedback with my doctor before I start using it?

A: You do not need to have it approved by your doctor; however, if you want your insurance to pay for it, you will need to ask him or her to consider it as adjunctive to your treatment. It might be a good idea to give him permission to discuss your case with your biofeedback therapist for a better understanding of your physiology and your problem.

Q: Will biofeedback hurt me in the long run?

A: You can be assured that biofeedback will help you in the long run. There are no negative sides of learning how to heal yourself. In fact, I believe that this training may be one of the best investments a person could make for their health in the future.

Q: Does biofeedback interact with any medications?

A: As a matter of fact, it is known that stress will interfere with medication usage by the body. Pain medicine is not as effective if the person is stressed. Insulin is not as effective, even antibiotics and anti-inflammatories, are not as effective under stress. When a patient releases his or her stress, the medications can have an enhanced impact.

Q: Are you certified or licensed in what you do?

A: I am a licensed psychologist and can perform biofeedback as part of my professional training. However, I would highly recommend training sponsored by the Association for Applied Psychophysiology and certification by the Biofeedback Certification Institute of America.

Q: How long did you go to school to do this?

A: I went to school for a lot of years (bachelors, masters, doctorate, plus residency and extended training) to learn to do what I do, but I do not confine myself just to biofeedback therapy. My approaches are very broad, especially since I am an old man and have done just about everything. If I were just starting out to be a biofeedback therapist, I would want to get a masters degree minimally, usually about six years of college past a high school education, but I would want to get as much information as I could about biology and the various models of health care.

Suggested Readings

Association for Applied Psychophysiology and Biofeedback. Available at: www.aapb.org

Biofeedback Certification Institute of America. Available at: www.bcia.org

Schwartz M, Andrasik F. *Biofeedback: A Practitioner's Guide*. 3rd ed. New York, NY: Guilford Press; 2003.

Robbins J. *A Symphony in the Brain: The Evolution of the New Brain Wave Biofeedback*. New York, NY: Grove Atlantic Inc; 2000.

Blumenstein B. *Brain and Body in Sport and Exercise: Biofeedback application in Performance Enhancement*. New York, NY: John Wiley and Sons; 2002.

References

1. Freeman L, Lawlis F. *Mosby Textbook for Complementary and Alternative Medicine: A Research-Based Approch*. St Louis, MO: Mosby; 2001.

11

Hypnosis

Daniel I. Galper, PhD

About the Author

Daniel I. Galper is a clinical psychologist and neuroscientist with specialized training in behavioral medicine. Dr. Galper's doctoral research at Virginia Tech examined psychological correlates of hypnotizability. As a post-doctoral clinical and National Institute of Health sponsored research fellow at the University of Virginia School of Medicine, Dr. Galper used hypnosis and biofeedback to assist patients with chronic pain, anxiety, cancer, obesity, diabetes, and various neurobehavioral problems. Dr. Galper is currently a senior research associate in the Department of Psychiatry at University of Texas Southwestern Medical Center at Dallas, and project director of the NIMH-funded Treatment with Exercise Augmentation for Depression (TrEAD) trial.

Q: What experience do you have with hypnosis?

A: I have been practicing clinical hypnosis since 1994 and conducting research on hypnosis and hypnotizability since 1995. During my doctoral studies in clinical psychology at Virginia Tech, I completed several courses in clinical and experimental hypnosis; I conducted research on the relation between hypnotizability and psychopathology in college students; and I read every book and journal article on hypnosis that I could get my hand on. I also was fortunate to be able to work with Dr. Helen J. Crawford, a cognitive neuroscientist at Virginia Tech, and one of the world's leading experts on the neurophysiology of hypnosis and hypnotic analgesia (pain control). As a graduate student in Dr. Crawford's laboratory, I assisted with a wide range of experimental studies examining cognitive and neural mechanisms of hypnosis, as well as behavioral and psychophysiological difference between low and highly hypnotizable individuals.[1,2] In 1998, I received an Erika Fromm and Milla Alihan Award from the Society for Clinical and Experimental Hypnosis for my research investigating associations between hypnotizability, dissociation, and abnormal eating in women.[3] I also completed post-doctoral clinical training and supervision in medical hypnosis at the University of Virginia School of Medicine and over 15 professional training workshops on ethical uses of hypnosis in medicine and psychotherapy.

In my clinical work, I have often used hypnosis to assist clients with a wide array of medical, neurobehavioral, and psychosocial problems, including acute and chronic pain, obesity, eating disorders, cancer, anxiety, psychological trauma, post-surgical recovery, and insomnia. I have also found hypnosis to be beneficial for smoking cessation and for enhancing concentration and performance in athletes and musicians. Finally, since 1997 I have provided hypnosis education and training to both medical and mental health professionals.

Q: What is hypnosis?

A: The term "hypnosis" is frequently used in reference to either 1) a psychological or mental state, or 2) a set of therapeutic techniques that are a type of "mind-body" medicine. With regard to the former, hypnosis is an alternate state of awareness characterized by observable changes in a person's behavior, perception, and cognition.[4,5] The behavioral changes may include alterations in physiological functions, such as respiration, autonomic activation (e.g., vagal/sympathetic balance), cellular immunity, cerebral blood flow, and brainwave activity, although the specific responses depend upon the hypnotic techniques used and the individual's level of hypnotizability. Interestingly, in support of the validity of hypnosis, some cognitive and physiological changes demonstrated under hypnosis are not reproducible by non-hypnotized persons trying to mimic or fake hypnosis.[1]

Hypnosis is often viewed as a passive condition, akin to muscular relaxation. Yet, we now know that hypnosis can be induced without relaxation.

For instance, several recent studies have examined the cognitive and neuro-physiological effects of hypnotic suggestions during aerobic and anaerobic exercise.[6] In addition, research shows that hypnosis actually involves increased effort and cerebral activation in several regions of the brain, although this effort may be dissociated from awareness.[1,2] Therefore, perhaps contrary to popular belief, hypnosis is a complex psychophysiological phenomenon, and it is not equivalent to physical relaxation, suggestion, or a placebo effect.

On the other hand, "hypnotic techniques" are the specific therapeutic procedures used by clinicians and researchers. These techniques include various types of hypnotic inductions and suggestions. In clinical practice, hypnotic techniques are used to alter or reframe patient behaviors, sensations, cognitions, and/or emotions. To maximize the therapeutic response, the specific hypnotic techniques are ideally tailored to each patient's needs, preferences, and goals.[7] Hypnotic inductions and suggestions have been shown to facilitate the effectiveness of various medical or psychological treatments.[8,9] For example, I often use hypnosis to enhance cognitive-behavioral psychotherapy and physiological self-regulation for men and women with phobias and post-traumatic stress disorder (PTSD). People with these anxiety disorders are often highly responsive to hypnosis,[10] and hypnosis can be applied to promote improved symptom control, as well as to facilitate cognitive restructuring and systematic desensitization. Because hypnosis can reduce physiological responses to stress[11,12] and increase neurobehavioral control, it can be an effective adjunctive treatment for obesity, smoking cessation, and neurobehavioral problems like irritable bowel syndrome and chronic pain.[5,8,9]

Q: Can everyone be hypnotized?

A: This question has been at the center of debate among clinicians and researchers in the field of hypnosis for many decades. Although some clinicians believe most everyone can be hypnotized, current research indicates that the ability to experience hypnosis, or one's hypnotizability, is a personality characteristic that lies within the individual. As I did in my research, a person's hypnotizability is easily assessed using special scales that measure the behavioral and subjective responses to standardized "test" suggestions.[13] In general, hypnotizability remains very stable over time, as indicated by a study at Stanford University showing a test-retest reliability of 0.71 over a 25-year period.[14] However, like other dimensions of personality, there is significant variability in hypnotizability within the general population: about two thirds of adults are moderate to highly responsive to hypnosis, while one third are basically non-responsive. In addition, children tend to be more hypnotizable than adults, and individuals with certain psychological disorders (e.g., anxiety, post-traumatic stress disorder, eating disorders, dissociative disorders) are often more hypnotizable. Although the reasons for such differences are not yet clear, there is evidence of fundamental biological and cognitive differences between low and highly hypnotizable persons. For instance, one recent study found highly hypnotizable individuals had a larger anterior corpus callosum,[2] a part of the brain responsible for the transfer of information between the two hemispheres within the frontal lobes, while other recent research points to genetic factors underlying individual differences in hypnotizability.[15]

Consistent with biological differences between low and highly hypnotizable individuals, current theories of hypnosis suggests that highly hypnotizable persons also possess a constellation of cognitive abilities different from less hypnotizable persons, including the ability to become deeply involved in experiences, to resist distractions, to flexibly access and regulate multiple levels of awareness, and to process some types of information automatically.[1,4] In addition, some studies have found highly hypnotizable individuals have more control over sleep processes[16] and report more intense emotional responses to positive and negative stimuli.[12]

Q: What is hypnosis like? Is hypnosis a normal experience?

A: Hypnotized persons often describe hypnosis as a condition of deeply involved and extremely focused concentration with activation of the imagination. As a person enters hypnosis, there is a reduction in awareness of reality and one's orientation to it, as well as increased access to internal sensations and experiences. In addition, hypnotized persons often demonstrate shifts in cognitive processing from more analytical and detail-oriented strategies during a normal alert state, to more holistic and imaginative strategies during hypnosis.[1,4] This is one reason why hypnosis is also believed to increase creativity and problem-solving in some situations.

A wide variety of experiences may occur during hypnosis different from normal waking consciousness. For instance, in my doctoral research I had the opportunity to hypnotize and observe hundreds of college students during imagined age regressions back to elementary school. Many of these subjects reported feeling as if they were 6 years old. In addition, many of these college students displayed handwriting similar to that of young children, with large sloppy letters and misspelled words. One woman who had studied French as a child, but since forgotten the language, actually wrote in French! When later interviewed about their experiences, these participants were usually surprised to see the dramatic changes in their handwriting, because the experience occurred outside of their awareness. Indeed, subjects often described their responses to hypnotic suggestions as relatively involuntary and automatic.

Thus, hypnosis involves fundamental shifts in information processing and working memory. Recent studies using advanced electroencephalogram and neuroimaging techniques also show dramatic shifts in functional neuroanatomy as hypnotizable persons enter hypnosis, with shifts in activation among neural structures implicated in executive processing, attention, emotion, homeostatic regulation, and visceral-sensory representation. I believe it is these changes in the hypnotized person's perception, behavior, and physiology that make hypnotic techniques particularly attractive and effective in clinical practice. On the other hand, hypnosis is also a very normal experience because it draws upon the innate cognitive resources of hypnotizable subjects. In fact, highly hypnotizable persons often report having "hypnotic-like" experiences, such as vivid images and alterations in time perception, outside of formal hypnosis.

Q: **What are some of the common myths and fears associated with hypnosis?**

A: There are many misconceptions regarding the nature of hypnosis. I have already noted that hypnosis is not the same as relaxation, although relaxation may be part of some hypnotic techniques. In addition, many people think that hypnosis will allow them to retrieve long forgotten childhood memories or locate misplaced objects. However, studies have demonstrated that information remembered through hypnosis is not more accurate than during normal recall. Thus, the only way to determine the true accuracy of material recalled under hypnosis is to obtain independent sources of corroboration. Furthermore, independent of the accuracy of memory, research has shown that hypnosis may falsely increase confidence in memories among highly hypnotizable persons. For this reason, some courts have refused to accept testimony that was remembered under hypnosis or after a person has been hypnotized. These issues are complex and beyond the scope of this discussion; however, they underscore the importance of receiving hypnosis only from professionals who are trained to understand and handle such issues.

The fear of "losing control" is perhaps the most common fear people have of hypnosis. People who have seen stage hypnosis may be afraid of embarrassing themselves under hypnosis or doing something they will later regret. This fear is related to the misbelief that hypnosis involves mind control or represents weak-mindedness. However, hypnotizability is not associated with gullibility, and hypnosis actually involves the utilization of ones own cognitive resources rather than the control of the hypnotist.

Q: **How do you decide whether to use hypnosis with a patient? How do you prepare a patient for using hypnosis?**

A: The clinical use of hypnosis depends upon many factors, the most important of which are the patient's motivation and openness to using hypnotic techniques, the patient's presenting symptoms, and the patient's hypnotizability.[5] Before using hypnosis, I always evaluate whether the patient is interested in hypnosis, his or her expectations for success, and whether hypnosis is likely to be useful in light of the clinical presentation.[7] Next, I educate the patient about hypnosis and clarify any fears and misconceptions, including those discussed earlier.[17] It is also important to instill positive expectations for success without being overly optimistic. Hypnotizability may be an important factor in the decision process, because it has been shown to predict treatment response. For instance, many studies have found that hypnotizability correlates with the degree of symptom reduction following hypnotic suggestions for pain relief. Obviously, highly hypnotizable individuals are most likely to benefit from hypnotic interventions. Less hypnotizable persons, particularly if highly motivated, may achieve some benefits from hypnosis; yet, other treatment approaches may be better suited to these individuals.

Q: What is a hypnotic induction? What are hypnotic suggestions?

A: Hypnotic inductions and suggestions are the most fundamental techniques in clinical hypnosis. Specifically, the induction is a set of verbal and non-verbal instructions and cues used by the clinician (or researcher) to capture the patient's attention, direct his intention, and prepare him or her for therapeutic change. During a hypnotic induction, which may last anywhere from 2–20 minutes (or more), depending on the situation, a transition occurs from the waking state into the hypnotic state, with consequent alternations in the individual's perception, behavior, and physiology, as discussed earlier. I closely observe each patient's responses to the induction, taking particular note of his or her posture, muscle tone, respiration, and affect.

Following the induction, hypnotic suggestions or other instructions may be used to help process or reframe the patient's cognitions, emotions, sensations, and/or physiological responses. Hypnotic suggestions may take many different forms, including direct verbal commands for particular responses and indirect images and metaphors for change or insight. These suggestions may be aimed at producing immediate effects within the hypnotic session or post-hypnotic responses, which are behavioral responses that occur at some time after hypnosis has been terminated. The particular suggestions utilized depend upon the patient's hypnotizability, age, level of maturity, and presenting problem, as well as the treatment goals. I often use laboratory equipment to monitor the patient's physiological response to hypnotic techniques to determine his level of engagement in the experience and potential to benefit from various hypnotic suggestions. Psychophysiological monitoring also allows me to tailor the hypnotic experience to maximize the probability for success.

Q: How does hypnosis work? What are the mechanisms of hypnosis?

A: Although the exact cognitive and neuropsychological mechanisms underlying hypnotic behavior and awareness are not fully understood, many cognitive and neuroscientific studies suggest that the frontal lobes of the brain, and particularly the pre-frontal and anterior cingulate cortices, direct downward control of lower neural centers that regulate emotion, autonomic function, sensory perception and representation. Indeed, activation of the frontal lobes and related limbic and brainstem structure of the brain, as well as shifts in cerebral activation and function, have often been found in highly hypnotizable persons following hypnotic inductions and suggestions.[1,4,6,16] Furthermore, hypnosis may enhance psychotherapy by intensifying the doctor–patient relationship. However, the mechanisms through which hypnotic suggestions are transformed by the brain/body into perceptual and physiological changes are not yet known and may never be fully understood.

Q: Can a person hypnotize himself or herself?

A: Yes, it is possible to hypnotize yourself. In fact, because hypnosis depends upon the abilities of the patient, most hypnosis experts believe that all hypnosis is really self-hypnosis. In practice, self-hypnosis is essentially the same as hypnosis induced by a clinician or researcher, except the induction is provided via audiotape or through the subject's recall of a hypnotic induction. In my experience, after a person has been hypnotized and becomes familiar with the process, he or she can usually learn to induce and practice self-hypnosis as a powerful form of self-regulation. I generally work with patients to develop self-hypnotic skills in therapy, and I encourage patients to practice self-hypnosis outside of their treatment sessions. Patients often report that regular practice of self-hypnosis increases their feelings of control and their coping abilities.

Q: Is hypnosis accepted as a valid therapeutic technique?

A: Hypnosis is widely considered a valid clinical technique (or as I view it a set of techniques), and hypnosis has played an important role over the centuries in psychotherapy, medicine and, more recently, in neuroscience. Hypnosis is approved by the American Medical Association, the British Medical Association, and the American Psychological Association. In addition, both clinical trials and meta-analyses have documented the efficacy of hypnosis from a wide range of problems.

Q: What healthcare problems can hypnosis benefit? How effective is hypnosis?

A: Although hypnosis is not a magic bullet and is not effective for everyone, hypnotic techniques can be extremely effective for some clinical problems. In my experience, hypnosis tends to be most effective for anxiety reduction, as well as the management of stress, acute and chronic pain, and the side effects of cancer chemotherapy, like nausea and vomiting.

In the 19th century, James Esdaile, MD,[18] used of hypnosis as the sole anesthetic for literally hundreds of minor and major surgeries in India. Interestingly, he observed that many of his patients showed increased resistance to infection, highlighting the potential effects of hypnosis on the immune system, a topic of on-going research.[11] More recently, following the pioneering work of the Hilgards at Stanford University in the 1960s, 70s, and 80s,[1,13] many studies have documented the benefits of hypnosis for pain and related symptoms.[9] This research suggests that hypnosis can often reduce pain, even when conventional treatments have failed. Furthermore, hypnosis has a number of advantages over other conventional and non-conventional techniques for pain control because it is non-invasive and easily applied in a variety of inpatient and outpatient settings, including the emergency room, with minimal preparation. In addition, there is evidence that hypnosis may be particularly beneficial for individuals with irritable bowel syndrome, eating disorders, dental procedures, weight-loss and smoking cessation.

Q: What research has been done on hypnosis?

A: There continues to be a tremendous amount of research on hypnosis, although the quality varies considerably. Some of the best hypnosis research is currently playing a key role in unraveling important links between the mind and body, as well as the neural pathways that control sensory perception, cognition, emotion, and pain. There are several peer-reviewed journals specifically devoted to hypnosis, including the *International Journal of Clinical and Experimental Hypnosis*, *American Journal of Clinical Hypnosis*, and *Contemporary Hypnosis*. Furthermore, hypnosis research is increasingly published in many of the leading journals in medicine, psychology, psychiatry, and neuroscience. Hypnosis studies range from those focusing on the subjective experience and how it compares to other states of consciousness, to experimental studies on cognitive and neurological factors that underlie differences in hypnotizability, to randomized clinical trials examining the effects of hypnosis on various clinical disorders, to name three.

Q: How much does hypnosis cost? Does insurance reimburse you for it?

A: Hypnosis is never used in isolation from a primary medical or psychological treatment. Hence, the cost of hypnosis depends on the cost of the primary treatment. For instance, one session of psychotherapy may cost between $50 to $250, with or without adjunctive hypnosis. Some insurance carriers specifically cover the cost of hypnosis, while others do not.

Q: What are the risks associated with hypnosis?

A: The large majority of people describe hypnosis as very pleasant, and negative responses are rare, although some presenting problems require a high degree of clinical skill when working with hypnosis. The only contraindications to hypnosis are poor clinical training, poor preparation and debriefing of the patient, and weak therapeutic boundaries.[17] Although hypnosis is generally very safe when used in an ethical manner, there have been cases where hypnosis was used to coerce patients. The actual role of hypnosis in these cases is not known and is a topic of some debate. It bears noting that some highly hypnotizable individuals may be vulnerable to this type of manipulation by an unethical clinician.

Q: How do I find someone qualified to use hypnosis?

A: The best way to find a qualified practitioner of hypnosis is to contact one of the three main professional hypnosis organizations, namely the American Society of Clinical Hypnosis (ASCH), the Society for Clinical and Experimental Hypnosis (SCEH), and Division 30 (Psychological Hypnosis) of the American Psychological Association (APA). Each of these organizations can provide a list of referrals and their qualifications. I would also like to give a word of caution regarding lay hypnotists who are not licensed healthcare providers and do not have adequate clinical training to handle the range of situations that may occur in clinical practice.[17]

Q: Will my doctor approve of hypnosis? Do I need to contact my doctor before I start using hypnosis?

A: Although hypnosis is often effective, few physicians have training in clinical hypnosis, and it is currently under utilized in clinical practice. Unfortunately, most doctors are unlikely to suggest hypnosis except in a final attempt to help a patient who has failed to respond to conventional therapies. Many physicians are learning about the potential benefits of hypnosis and are supportive of patients who want to try hypnosis. In my clinical work at the University of Virginia School of Medicine, I provided hypnotic interventions to patients from various clinics throughout the hospital. Although many physicians were initially skeptical about hypnosis, most began to appreciate the benefits hypnosis provided to their patients.

As with any clinical practice with the potential to alter one's physiology and health, it is generally important to inform your doctor about your intention to use hypnosis. It is also a good idea to keep your doctor informed regarding your treatment progress, as this may affect other treatment recommendations.

Q: How can I learn more about hypnosis?

A: A few graduate and medical schools offer courses and supervision in clinical and experimental hypnosis. Most practitioners learn hypnosis by attending training workshops sponsored by the ASCH, SCEH, and the APA. Information on hypnosis workshops and other resources offered through these organizations can be found on the Internet. I encourage clinicians to attain training through one of these organizations rather than through one of the many online "schools" offering "hypnotherapy."*

---

* This chapter was developed with support from a NARSAD Young Investigator Award to Dr. Galper, and NIH (NCCAM) grant T32-AT-00052.

References

1. Crawford HJ. Brain dynamics and hypnosis: Attentional and disattentional processes. *Int J Clin Exp Hypn.* 1994;42:204–232.

2. Horton JE, Crawford HJ, Harrington G, Downs JH. Increased anterior corpus callosum size associated positively with hypnotizability and the ability to control pain. *Brain.* 2004;127:1741–1747.

3. Galper DI, Crawford HJ. Disordered eating in college women: To what degree are dissociation, hypnotizability, and attentional styles of relevance? Paper presented at the 49th Annual Scientific Sessions of the Society for Clinical and Experimental Hypnosis, Chicago, IL. November 1998.

4. Crawford HJ, Brown AM, Moon CE. Sustained attentional and disattentional abilities: Differences between low and highly hypnotizable persons. *J Abnorm Psychol* 1993;102:534–543.

5. Galper DI. Hypnosis. In: Wren K, Norred C, eds. *Real World Nursing Survival Guide: Complementary and Alternative Therapies.* Philadelphia, PA: Saunders; 2003:152–156.

6. Williamson JW, McColl R, Mathews D, Mitchell, JH, Raven PB, Morgan WP. Hypnotic manipulation of effort sense during dynamic exercise: cardiovascular responses and brain activation. *J App Physiol.* 2001;90:1392–1399.

7. Kessler RS, Dane JR, Galper DI. Conversational assessment of hypnotic ability to promote hypnotic responsiveness. *Am J Clin Hypn.* 2002:44:273–282.

8. Kirsch I, Montgomery G, Sapirstein G. Hypnosis as an adjunct to cognitive-behavioral psychotherapy: a meta-analysis. *J Consult Clin Psychol.* 1995;63:214–220.

9. Montgomery GH, Duhamel KN, Redd WH. A meta-analysis of hypnotically induced analgesia: how effective is hypnosis? *Int J Clin Exp Hypn.* 2000;48:138–153.

10. Bryant RA, Guthrie RM, Moulds ML. Hypnotizability and acute stress disorder. *Am J Psychiatry, 158.* 2001;158:600–604.

11. Kiecolt-Glaser JK, Marucha PT, Atkinson C, Glaser R. Hypnosis as a modulator of cellular immune dysregulation during acute stress. *J Consult Clin Psychol.* 2001;69:674–682.

12. Zachariae R, Jørgensen MM, Bjerring P, Svendsen G. Autonomic and psychological responses to an acute psychological stressor and relaxation: the influence of hypnotizability and absorption. *Int J Clin Exp Hypn.* 2000; 48:388–403.

13. Hilgard ER. *Hypnotic Susceptibility.* New York, NY: Harcourt, Brace, & World; 1965.

14. Piccione C, Hilgard ER, Zimbardo P. On the degree of stability of measured hypnotizability over a 25-year period. *J Pers Soc Psychol.* 1989;56:289–295.

15. Lichtenberg P, Bachner-Malman R, Ebstein RP, Crawford HJ. Hypnotic susceptibility: multidimensional relationships with Cloninger's Tridimensional Personality Questionnaire, COMT polymorphisms, absorption, and attentional charistics. *Int J Clin Exp Hypn.* 2004;52:47–72.

16. Evans FJ. Hypnotizability: individual differences in dissociation and the flexible control of psychological processes. In: Lynn SJ, Rhue JW, eds. *Theories of Hypnosis: Current Models and Perspectives*. New York, NY: Guilford Press; 1991:144–168.

17. Crawford HJ, Kitner-Triolo M, Clark SW, Olesko B. Transient positive and negative experiences accompanying stage hypnosis. *J Abnorm Psychol* 1992;101: 663–667.

18. Esdaile J. *Hypnosis in Medicine and Surgery: The Work of James Esdaile, M.D.* New York, NY: The Julian Press; 1957.

12

Music Therapy and the Effects of Music

Heather A. Schmidt, PhD, DM, MA

About the Author

Heather A. Schmidt is an internationally renowned concert pianist and composer. She has performed throughout North America and in many countries abroad including Germany, France, the Czech Republic, Iceland, Finland, Brazil, Mexico, and the British West Indies. Her many accolades include three BMI awards and a Juno nomination in the category of "Best Classical Composition." As an educator and teacher, she frequently lectures on topics related to music and health. In addition to a musical education that includes studies at Juilliard and a Doctor of Music degree from Indiana University, she also holds a MA in Psychology. She is the founder and executive director of the Optimal Performance Institute, a nonprofit entity that seeks to promote health in musicians and health through music. For more information, please visit her website available at **www.heatherschmidt.com.**

Q: What got you interested in the effects of music and music therapy?

A: Music has had a very strong impact on my life from an early age. I began piano lessons at the age of 4 and I loved classical music instantly. I went on to study at Juilliard and became a professional concert pianist and composer. Over time, I have become increasingly interested in the effects of music on health, and in the relationships between music and various aspects of psychology and emotion, including the benefits of listening to music and the field of music therapy. While maintaining an active career as a professional musician, I have pursued graduate studies in psychology and I continue to develop my interest in researching the relationships between music and health.

Q: Why do you believe in the healing potential of music?

A: As a musician, I have personally had the opportunity to witness the profound effects of music upon musicians and non-musicians alike. As a performer and composer, I regularly travel throughout North America and abroad and my frequent travels have enabled me to interact with musicians and audiences in many different contexts. I have seen people experience significant emotional and physiological changes as they listened to music. Historical and scientific literature provides countless examples of cases where people's psychological and physical states have been altered through music. The practice of healing through music dates back to ancient times, and has been explored in many different cultures.

Q: What is music therapy?

A: Music therapy is a diverse field, in which music is used as a treatment method to enhance health and to elicit emotional, physiological, behavioral, and/or social changes. Music therapy is highly tailored to each situation and the exact nature of the treatment plan varies according to the specific needs of each individual.

Q: In what context is music therapy used?

A: Music therapy is used in a wide variety of settings including hospitals, schools, nursing homes, and mental health facilities. Among other situations, music therapy is used as a treatment method for populations that are affected by physical disabilities, mental disorders, developmental disabilities, learning disorders, communication disorders, behavioral disorders, social disorders, and post-traumatic stress disorders. Music therapy may also be used as a pre- and post-surgical intervention, as an adjunct to assist childbirth and labor, and as a technique for pain management and stress and anxiety reduction. People in good health without a specific ailment may also benefit from music therapy through its promotion of relaxation, creativity, and intellectual stimulation. Individuals of all ages may benefit from music therapy, from premature babies to the elderly. Outside of music therapy, music is also incorporated into the treatment methods of practitioners in other professional fields, including psychology and psychophysiology.

Q: What are the benefits of music and music therapy?

A: Music and music therapy offer many potential benefits including relaxation and stress reduction, positive changes in mood and emotional state, heightened creativity, intellectual stimulation and development, and positive changes in physiology.

Components of physiology that may be altered through music include heart rate, muscle tension, respiration rate, blood pressure, blood volume, skin temperature, hormone secretion, endorphin release, and immune function.

Q: What does music therapy involve and how does it work?

A: The field of music therapy is extremely diverse and music therapy can involve a variety of different treatment methods. Although all of the exact mechanisms are not fully understood, emotional and physiological changes through music have been identified in numerous clinical and research settings. Simply listening to music can evoke emotional and physiological changes. Music therapy often involves listening to music specifically chosen to evoke particular emotional and physical responses. Although no musical ability or training is required on the part of any client seeking music therapy, certain treatment methods within music therapy may involve some form of active participation in a musical activity. This musical participation can affect the client's emotional and physiological state, as well as his or her behaviors and social skills. Musical participation can also increase creativity and intellectual development. In situations seeking to promote behavioral or social modification (such as in cases of clients with autism, developmental disability, or mental health disorder), music may be introduced or withdrawn as reinforcement to encourage appropriate social or behavioral modification.

Q: Is research available that supports the effectiveness of music therapy?

A: A significant quantity of research has examined music therapy and the effects of music. Much of this research supports the efficacy of music therapy in a variety of contexts. The body of research on topics related to music and music therapy continues to expand annually, and there are many different types of research being conducted in these areas. For example, research projects range from studies about the effects of music therapy on a specific disorder such as Alzheimer's disease or autism, to research examining the effects of specific kinds of music on different populations in different settings. There are a number of journals devoted exclusively to the profession of music therapy including the *Journal of Music Therapy* and *Music Therapy Perspectives*. A large volume of scientific research involving music has been done in the fields of psychology, psychophysiology, neuroscience, and neurophysiology. Many topics within these larger research areas are directly or indirectly related to music therapy.

Q: How many people practice music therapy as a profession?

A: The practice of music therapy is widespread in the United States, Canada, and in a number of European countries including Sweden and France. The largest professional association of music therapy is the American Music Therapy Association that has over 5000 members. The lists of music therapists do not include the many trained professionals in other disciplines who incorporate music into their practices.

Q: What type of training is involved to become a music therapist?

A: In North America, most music therapists receive undergraduate and/or graduate degrees in music therapy from an accredited degree program approved by the American Music Therapy Association. After completing an internship, music therapists complete a national examination through the Certification Board for Music Therapists. Continuation of a music therapist's certification is contingent upon continuing education and/or additional testing. Psychologists and other professionals who utilize music as a treatment method receive training in their respective disciplines through their degree programs, internships, post-doctoral training, seminars, and continuing education.

Q: How much does music therapy cost and does insurance reimburse you for it?

A: Due to the diversity and frequent changes in insurance policies, you should check with your individual provider to learn the details of allowable coverage. Music therapy is sometimes incorporated as a component of broader therapeutic and clinical treatments, and your insurance may be able to cover music therapy within these contexts. Costs for music therapy vary depending on the practitioner and the type of treatment involved. You should consult music therapists in your area for current rates.

Q: What will my doctor think of music therapy, and do I need my doctor's approval before starting music therapy?

A: It is always a good idea to consult with your doctor before beginning any new treatments. Music therapy is generally considered to be a form of treatment within complementary and alternative medicine, and it is often used simultaneously as an adjunct to conventional medical treatments. Although there is research supporting the efficacy of music therapy as a treatment modality,[1,2] medical doctors vary in their approval of treatments within the realm of complementary and alternative medicine. Should you decide to explore music therapy or other alternative medicine treatments, you may wish to consult a medical doctor who is open to the possibilities of alternative medicine and who is knowledgeable about these areas. Questions specific to music therapy can be answered by contacting music therapists in your area or by calling the American Association of Music Therapy for direction. If you notice that you are positively affected by music, either by listening passively or by actively engaging in a musical activity, you may benefit from incorporating music more frequently into your life on a personal basis, independently of a specific music therapy program.

Q: Are there any contraindications to music therapy?

A: The only potential contraindication to music therapy is a negative emotional or physiological response that arises as a reaction to a specific piece or style of music. Music has the potential to elicit powerful emotional responses, positive and negative, and an individual may be affected by the inherent qualities of certain types of music. In addition to the direct impact of the music itself, it is common for a specific piece of music to become closely tied to a strong positive or negative memory of an experience that occurred in proximity to when the piece of music was heard. Consequently, music associated with positive experiences can trigger positive feelings and the reverse is true for negative experiences. For instance, a recently divorced person may feel sadness or become upset when hearing a song that he or she listened to regularly with their former spouse. Negative reactions to music are generally mild and transient and they can often be prevented by avoiding music that provokes negative feelings either directly or through association. Personal preferences in music are highly individual and anyone seeking music therapy as a treatment should inform their music therapist of their preferences and alert their therapist regarding any specific music that may have negative personal associations. Music therapists are trained to inquire about individual preferences before selecting music for a particular client and they are also trained to notice signs in the client's behavioral or emotional state that indicate the effectiveness of a particular type of music.

Q: How will I know if music therapy is working for me, and how do I know if the effects I experience are from the music therapy and not from something else I am doing?

A: If you feel better and experience positive results through music therapy, it is likely that music therapy is working for you. It may be that the music therapy itself is responsible, or the benefits may be the combined result of music therapy synergistically with other things you are doing. When trying a variety of treatments simultaneously, it is difficult to isolate the effectiveness of music therapy alone unless you carefully control every other activity and compare them individually. It would seem reasonable to assume that the music therapy is a contributing factor to the benefits if you feel more improvements during and after music therapy than you did before you started. Medical measurements of your physiology before, during, and after music therapy can give you a more specific and tangible indication of how profoundly a particular physiological symptom is affected by music.

Q: Where can I find out more about music therapy and the effects of music?

A: The Internet is one of the best sources for up-to-date information on music research. Many books and articles are available, and you can find these items by checking your local libraries, bookstores, or by searching on-line. For specific information about music therapy, a good starting place is the American Music Therapy Association available at **www.musictherapy.org**. The importance of music for children, and other topics related to music and health, are available at **www.OptimalPerformanceInstitute.com**.

Q: What are the effects of just listening to music?

A: There are many potential benefits to listening to music. Listening to music can increase relaxation and it can enhance a positive mood. Many people find that they exercise more frequently or more effectively if they listen to music while they exercise. For some people, listening to music in the background can increase work productivity. Many children and adults with Attention Deficit Disorder or Attention Deficit Hyperactive Disorder find that they can concentrate better and work with more focused attention when music is playing in the background at a low volume. Listening to classical music such as Mozart may have additional benefits. The so-called "Mozart effect" refers to the positive effects of listening to Mozart's music.[3] The benefits of the Mozart Effect include improvement on spatial performance tasks and long-term improvements of spatial-temporal abilities in children.[4] Various neurophysiological changes in the brain also appear to result from exposure to Mozart's music.[5,6]

Q: How can I tell if listening to music is good for me?

A: You can determine how significantly music affects you by making subjective observations while listening to music. You can also consult music therapists and other related professionals for an external objective perspective. The more you expose yourself to different music, the more easily you can determine which kinds of music make you feel best.

Q: What are the effects of taking music lessons and learning to play an instrument?

A: Playing a musical instrument or singing can have the same effect as listening to music plus some additional benefits. Learning to play an instrument can promote creativity, improve and develop motor coordination, and stimulate intellectual development. Playing an instrument or singing can also serve as an effective emotional release. Belonging to a band, orchestra, chamber group, or choir can enhance the enjoyment of music in a social setting. A number of positive effects have been reported in children who take music lessons.[7,8] Youngsters with music training have been found to score higher on spatial-temporal testing and in certain areas of mathematics, including fractions.[9] Some studies have shown that music lessons during childhood actually enlarge the brain in certain areas, specifically the corpus callosum.[10,11] According to The College Board's 1998 Profiles of SAT and Achievement Test Takers, high school seniors who had music training in school scored significantly higher on SATs in both the verbal and math sections.[12] Students involved in music have been reported to have lower lifetime levels of substance abuse.[13]

Q: Is there a difference in the benefits of music depending upon what kind of music I listen to, and are certain types of music "better" than others?

A: Musical preferences vary significantly among individuals, and music that evokes a particular response from one person may have the completely opposite effect with another person. All music has the potential to elicit emotional and physiological changes, and individual responses and preferences will determine what types of music are "best" for each individual. It can be helpful to listen to a wide variety of musical styles, including music that you would not ordinarily choose. Some people limit themselves to a specific style of music and they are often surprised when they have a positive reaction to unfamiliar music that is not on their list of favorites.

To date, the majority of research indicates that the benefits of the Mozart effect occur only in music by Mozart and other similar classical music.[6,14] Non-classical music, including contemporary pop music, does not appear to create the stimulating benefits of classical music, possibly because the simplicity, shorter patterns and extensive repetition do not engage the brain in a comparable fashion. The Mozart effect phenomenon appears to occur in animals as well as humans. In one study, rats were exposed to one of four auditory conditions and tested for spatial-temporal ability in a maze. The four auditory conditions were: Mozart; a simple, repetitive piece by Philip Glass; silence; or white noise. The rats exposed to Mozart performed significantly better than the rats exposed to any of the other three conditions.

Q: Is there a difference between going to a live music performance and just listening to a recording?

A: There is an enormous difference between going to a live music performance versus just listening to a recording. Although recorded music has certain benefits and conveniences, live music performances have the capacity to touch, inspire, and excite on an entirely different level. The thrill of watching a live performer and experiencing the active communication between performers and audience cannot be adequately replicated in any audio or video format. The charisma and personality of a performer cannot be fully experienced in any way other than a live performance. In addition, there is some evidence that the social and cultural stimulation of live performance events may have a positive effect on health and wellness.

References

1. DeLoach WD. Procedural-support music therapy in the healthcare setting: a cost-effectiveness analysis. *J Pediatr Nurs.* 2005;20(4):276–284.

2. Gerdner LA. Use of individualized music by trained staff and family: translating research into practice. *J Gerontol Nurs.* 2005;31(6):22–30.

3. Rauscher FH, Shaw GL. Key components of the Mozart effect. *Percept Mot Skills.* 1998;86(3):835–841.

4. Bodner M, Muftuler LT, Nalcioglu O, Shaw GL. MRI study relevant to the Mozart effect: brain areas involved in spatial-temporal reasoning. *Neurol Res.* 2001;23(7):683–690.

5. Jenkins JS. The Mozart effect. *J R Soc Med.* 2001;94(4):170–172.

6. Jausovec N, Habe K. The "Mozart effect": an electroencephalographic analysis employing the methods of induced event-related desynchronization/synchronization and event-related coherence. *Brain Topogr.* 2003;16(2):73–84.

7. Overy K. Dyslexia and music. From timing deficits to musical intervention. *Ann N Y Acad Sci.* 2003;

8. Shahin A, Roberts, LE, Trainor LJ. Enhancement of auditory cortical development by musical experience in children. *NeuroReport.* 20041;5(12):1917–1921.

9. Cheek JM, Smith LR. Music training and mathematics achievement. *Adolescence.* 1999;34(136):759–761.

10. Myskja A, Lindbaek M. How does music affect the human body? *Tidssk Nor Laegeforen.* 2000;120(10):1182–1185.

11. Watkins GR. Music therapy: proposed physiological mechanisms and clinical implications. *Clin Nurse Spec.* 1997;11(2):43–50.

12. Schellenberg EG. Music lessons enhance IQ. *Psychol Sci.* 2004;15(8):511–514.

13. Harrison PA, Narayan G. Differences in behavior, psychological factors, and environmental factors associated with participation in school sports and other activities in adolescence. *J Sch Health.* 2003;73(3):113–120.

14. Steele KM. Arousal and mood factors in the "Mozart effect." *Percept Mot Skills.* 2000;91(1):188–190.

13

Yoga

Matthew J. Taylor, PhD, PT, RYT

About the Author

Matthew J. Taylor is a physical therapist and senior yoga therapist with 24 years of experience. In addition to his integrative private practice in Scottsdale, Arizona, he has created an online learning community of physical rehabilitation professionals that is available at **www.dynamicsystemsrehab.com**. More information is available at **www.myrehab.com**. He is completing his dissertation on a yoga-based back school for people with chronic spine pain, serves as a medical advisor to the International Association of Yoga Therapists, and continues to teach across the country.

Q: What is yoga anyway?

A: It is important to understand that our Western experience of yoga is typically a commercialized version of the ancient practice. Traditionally yoga's primary function was to create health or wholeness through the rediscovery of the yoked reality of life (yoga is derived from the Sanskrit verb "yuj," which means to yoke or join). We see this concept extolled in the modern-day marketing of "body, mind, and spirit." The traditional focus of yoga as a psycho-spiritual technology is on controlling the *fluctuations* of the mind, with the physical body serving as just one tool toward that end. The modern fixation on the physical outcomes of flexibility, balance, and physical health were considered secondary to having attained control of one's mind and subsequent spiritual development.

Q: What got you interested in yoga?

A: My physical therapy clinic has an integrated health club. One of my members suggested I invite a local yoga teacher to teach at our facility. I was intrigued from both a physical performance perspective and by the general health benefits of yoga. I also recognized yoga as an emerging fitness trend and believed it was a prudent business decision. What ignited my enthusiasm for the practice was when, as a highly skilled orthopedic physical therapist, I experienced healing of my own degenerating, chronic lower back condition. This occurred through a group yoga class with no treatment per se. That got my attention!

Q: In what ways do you have knowledge about yoga?

A: I will answer the question in **Table 13.1** from the metaperspectives of the interrelationship of my four ways of *knowing* yoga. The table also makes a template or tool for professionals to broaden their own "knowing/belief" inquiry into all forms of Complementary and Alternative Medicine (CAM).

Q: Does yoga really work?

A: Good question. Yoga by its 5000-year longevity suggests that something about yoga *works*. The yogic health model is one of a complex, dynamic living system. Because of that, no one can predict a specific outcome from any one individual starting a yoga class. Be sure to read the preceding and following questions for greater understanding.

Q: How does yoga work?

A: The yoga model of health is based on the optimal development of the whole human to include themselves and their communities. Yoga is far more than "stretching." A regular practice of all eight paths of yoga as depicted in **Table 13.2** provides for that optimal development.

Table 13.1 Ways of Knowing

Ways of Knowing	Definition/ Examples	My Knowing about Yoga
Propositional	Knowing in conceptual terms which are descriptions of reality through the language of statements, logic, and various propositions based on presentational forms traditionally in papers, theories, and hypotheses.	From my studies of medicine, biological dynamics systems, and integrative medicine I can propose coherent, logical formulations of how yoga supports healing and health.
Experiential	Knowing, which means the inquirer's direct encounter through participation; feeling and imaging the presence of some entity, person, place, energy, process, or thing.	Through my ongoing inquiry in the practice of yoga my chronic back condition is healed along with multiple other facets of my health.
Presentational	Knowing is grounded on images from experiential knowing. Described as an intuitive grasp of the significance of their experience of their world, it is symbolized in graphic, plastic, musical, vocal, and verbal-art forms.	How I write, speak, teach, and practice in the clinic is all radically changed and accomplished with much less effort. This chapter, and this table in fact, are examples of my presentational knowing of yoga.
Practical	Knowing is demonstrating a skill or competency. The ability to act in purposive deeds based on the other three forms of knowing culminates in practical skills from action.	Otherwise known as "outcomes." I move, live, and practice more effectively, more efficiently, and more compassionately than I did before I began my yoga practice.

The yoga health model proposes a person is made up of five interdependent and interrelated aspects known as "koshas" as outlined in **Table 13.3**. Practicing the eight paths has effects on all of the koshas. Amazingly, this 4000-year-old model describes the complexity offered in modern day dynamic systems theories of health (e.g., a back strain can ruin your mood, or depression can tighten up your back, or your creativity can be stymied by a sore back). It is all connected and interrelated.

Table 13.2 Patanjali's Eight-Fold Path

Path	Description
Yama	Moral precepts: non-harming, truthfulness, non-stealing, chastity, greedlessness
Niyama	Qualities to nourish: purity, contentment, austerity (exercise), self-study, devotion
Asana	A calm, firm steady stance in relation to life
Pranayama	The ability to channel and direct breath and life energy
Pratyahara	Focusing on senses inward; non-reactivity to stimuli
Dharana	Concentration
Dhyana	Meditation
Samadhi	Ecstatic union; flow; "in the zone"

Source: Taylor, MJ. *Integrating Yoga Therapy into Rehabilitation*. Galena, IL: Embug Publishing; 1999:14.

Table 13.3 Clinical Translations of the Koshas

Sanskrit	Common Name	Description
Anna-maya-kosha Body	Food Sheath	Comprised of the physical, solid aspect of a human (i.e. cells, organs, bones, joints, etc.)
Prana-maya-kosha Body	Life Force Sheath	The bioelectric forces and breath are a portion of prana. Similar to "Chi" or "Qi" concepts in Chinese medicine.
Mano-maya-kosha Mind	Thought/Primitive Mind Sheath	Includes emotions, reactive thinking, reflexes, or subcortical function; is largely shared with the rest of the animal kingdom.
Vijnana-maya-kosha Mind	Wisdom/Higher Mind Sheath	Includes the higher cortical functions of reflection, intuition, planning, and creativity; not as developed in animals.
Ananda-maya-kosha Spirit	Bliss Sheath	Sometimes equated to the soul or spirit of the patient.

Source: Taylor, MJ. *Integrating Yoga Therapy into Rehabilitation*. Galena, IL: Embug Publishing; 1999:22.

Q: How do I know if yoga is working and not something else I am doing?

A: I am afraid you cannot know for certain. Modern quantum and chaotic systems theory stress that *uncertainty* is the hallmark of today's medicine. I suggest back to you, if you are experiencing enhanced well being, *under your physician's guidance*, try modifying or eliminating the most noxious and expensive independent variables first. My experience has been that often modifications are possible *and* that yoga is generally among the least expensive and almost always carries the fewest negative side effects.

Q: Are there any consequences to my health?

A: The fruits of a proper yoga practice should be *sthira* and *sukha*, or "sweetness/ steadiness" and "calm/comfort." An ineffective practice by contrast leaves the individual agitated, angry, in pain, fearful, or otherwise. Such a state sustains a chronic stress response. The deleterious effects on health in such an environment are well documented. By contrast, the evidence is mounting for the positive health effects of the relaxation response of a proper practice that produces *sthira* and *sukha*.

Q: How many people use yoga?

A: The number of people using yoga continues to grow as the practice enjoys increasing popularity. Estimates range from 20–30 million up to 23% of the population of the United States practice yoga. Yoga is finding its way into the medical community through hospital-based wellness programs, cardiac rehab, and chronic pain management, as well as in physical education classes, health clubs, church health ministries, and retreat centers. The range of use varies from sitting quietly while attending to the breath for a few minutes to an intense 90-minute daily practice.

Q: What type of research has been done in yoga?

A: Most of the research done to date has been out of India. In the past decade the studies out of India have begun to adopt Western standards, and there have been a number of studies emerging out of Western universities as well. I work with people around the world on research projects and it is very exciting to see the new studies being undertaken. Further yoga research information is available at **www.yrec.org** and **www.yogatherapy.org**.

Q: What will my doctor think about this?

A: The actual initial response is not important. What is important is your or your patient's follow-up inquiry into the basis for your physician's thoughts. Your doctor's knowledge can range from an ungrounded biased opinion to a serious, well thought out medical concern. Follow-up questions to ask include asking about their experience, the specific reason such a practice would be contraindicated, and the possibility of modifying a practice under their guidance. A physician or any other healthcare provider who declines discussing your concerns or dismisses outright any CAM without thoughtful explanation may not be your best partner in managing your health.

Q: Do I need to approve yoga with my doctor before I start using it?

A: Certainly, if you are under a doctor's care or taking medications for a chronic illness. If you are not in good health, physically and mentally robust, and active the answer is less definite. One of the foundations of yoga is "ahimsa," or non-violence. My suggestion to people in this category of health is if you have a physician who knows your state of health, how can it do harm to ask? Finally, if your yoga instructor does not ask you a thorough medical screening questionnaire before your first instruction, think long and hard about continuing with that teacher.

Q: Does yoga interact with any of the medications I may be taking?

A: Yes. There are multiple interactions possible and you should discuss any changes in your experiences with both your instructor and your physician. The interactions can be either positive or negative. Bottom line: communicate regularly with both your physician and teacher *any* changes you are experiencing.

Q: What type of medical conditions can be supported by a yoga practice?

A: The only prerequisite for participating in yoga is active respiration. There are prenatal, postpartum, pediatric, children's, teen's, general adult, diagnosis specific, geriatric, and end-of-life transitional yoga programs. Yoga is very popular among athletes, performers, seniors, and aging boomers. There are programs for cardiac health, women's health, fall prevention, creativity, stress management, and chronic pain. Yoga is by definition the science of integration and healthy responses to life.

Q: How can I make time for yoga? I'm already too busy.

A: That is one of the wonderful paradoxes of practicing yoga: by taking time to practice you create more time in the rest of your day. There are a myriad of reasons for this phenomena that include
- Better quality of sleep and therefore requiring less sleep;
- Enhanced concentration for increased productivity;
- Clarity in priorities facilitates, *first things first*;
- Freedom from inauthentic commitments to "must haves or do's";
- Modified food consumption, selection, and portion control reduces the lethargy of overconsumption; and,
- A learned relaxation response permits faster, more effective recovery and restoration from fatigue and illness.

   Take the 4-week test: practice 30 minutes a day for 4 weeks. If you are not less harried, more productive and better rested, try something else.

Q: I am not very flexible, strong, or balanced. Can I still do yoga?

A: Yes. The books filled with pictures of people in all forms of contortion represent the "Olympians" of yoga. Your instructor will work with you from where you are now in regards to your mobility, flexibility, and strength. The standard of yoga is an *internal* focus on where you are right now, looking neither into the future, the past, and most especially, not across the room at someone else! The "ego" portion of the mind will constantly disrupt (*fluctuate*) with judgments, memories, or rehearsals ("I'm too tight," "She's so good," "If I push a little harder I'll touch the floor," etc.). When you catch yourself in this mode, congratulations. It is the first step toward the goal of yoga: controlling the fluctuations of the mind!

Q: Doesn't yoga hurt?

A: Another definition of yoga is transformation. Anytime a human being undergoes growth or change in transformation there will be varying degrees of "discomfort" physically, emotionally, psychically, and spiritually. The discomfort arises from the resistance of the ego portion of the mind fearing loss of its identity and control. This is where having an experienced and compassionate teacher is critical. They can modify your practice, offer suggestions and support, or make appropriate referrals if need be.

Q: I am a conservative Christian, Jew, Muslim, etc. Can I still do yoga and not compromise my religious tradition?

A: Yoga is a spiritual science, but makes no specific statement about a belief in God or deities. By spiritual, I mean it examines the big questions of self-conscious human inquiry: Who am I?, What am I?, and What or how shall I act or be in this reality? By contrast a traditional religious practice offers answers to these questions, while a person's spiritual practice confirms those answers through experience and self-reflection. Yoga arose out of the Hindu, Jain, and Buddhist religious traditions and draws on some of their concepts but makes no dogmatic demands of belief in any specific deity or other expression of spirituality. Yoga is a spiritual path that has been practiced and adapted by people of all creeds.

Q: Isn't yoga just another New Age fad?

A: No, the New Age movement has embraced elements of yoga, most noticeably those that are trendy or create dramatic sensations or experiences. However, sincere practitioners of yoga recognize yoga as a still evolving philosophical science of self. As such, the 5000-year-old tradition is honored and preserved while it grows and changes today.

Q: Do I have to be a vegetarian, wear funny clothes, or do strange things to practice yoga?

A: No, yoga requires no specific external changes in behavior or appearance. No funny clothes, toe rings, or hairdos. As the student develops the discipline of the mind and responds to life proactively with authentic self-awareness, inevitably there will be practical changes in behavior. One's diet may be modified, or you might decline chemical lawn treatments, or adopt a more sustainable pattern of consumption. The most dramatic changes are interior changes that manifest in a more tolerant, strong, and flexible human being.

Q: Can you help me understand all the various types of yoga I hear about?

A: Confusion develops around the various types of yoga because in our culture of brand identification the traditional category of yoga, teacher lineages, and blended business names has generated a myriad of types. Please see the recommended resources at the conclusion of this chapter for a detailed explanation. Hatha yoga is the most popular and prevalent type of yoga in the West. Hatha yoga is a subcategory of the Hindu yoga tradition, which along with other categories such as Raja, Bhakti, Laya, Karma, and Jnana compose one hierarchical level of classification. Under hatha there are then descending levels of classification mixed by teacher, lineage, and brand name. Consider the following fictitious yoga studio in your hometown as a frame of reference for asking questions of yoga instructors, which with the references, will allow you to then determine if it is a type of yoga suitable for your needs (see **Table 13.4**).

Q: Do you have to be certified or licensed to teach yoga?

A: No, in the United States there are presently no regulations or certifications governing yoga teachers. There is a national teacher's registry, Yoga Alliance (available at **www.yogaalliance.org**) that has basic minimum standards for schools and individual teachers. It is a voluntary program that entitles the teacher to use RYT (Registered Yoga Teacher) after their name and offers the public some assurance of the individual having participated in a training program. However, there is no testing and the registry makes no assertions of competency. There is a wide variance in teacher training

Table 13.4 Types of Yoga

What tradition do you teach?	Does your yoga have a common classification?	What is your teacher lineage?	What school or style do you teach from?	What is the name of your business?
Hindu Yoga Tradition	Hatha Yoga	Krishnama-charya and B.K. Iyengar	Iyengar School of Yoga	BunsOSteel Yoga

ranging from no training to the true master instructors who have earnestly lived and studied the practice for over 30 or 40 years. The bottom line is due diligence is required by both a referring medical practitioner and the individual consumer. Phone interviews with teachers, sampling classes, and checking references are recommended as minimum prudent risk management action steps prior to beginning instruction.

On a related note, at this time there is legally no such thing as a "yoga therapist." From the legal standpoint, all yoga therapy is merely instruction in yoga. Otherwise, yoga therapy as a therapeutic modality would warrant governmental regulation. But remember, because all yoga instruction is intended to facilitate a rediscovery of wholeness, by definition all yoga is therapeutic.

Q: How long did you go to school to do this?

A: I have over 500 hours of training in yoga instruction with an emphasis on supporting medically challenged clients. I am also completing 48 doctoral hours at the California Institute of Integral Studies in preparation for my dissertation in a yoga-based program with an emphasis on transformational learning and change (yoga). My dissertation will be yoga based and I continue to write articles for professional journals around the world. I teach medical professionals across the country how to use yoga in traditional settings and constantly learn from them as well.

Q: How much does yoga cost?

A: There is a wide variance in charges dependent upon the setting, type of instruction, and instructor. A group yoga class taught in a yoga studio by a yoga teacher will run somewhere from $10 to $20 per class. Individual yoga instruction can run from $50 on up to between $100 and $200 per hour from a renowned or very experienced teacher. When delivered as a prescribed therapeutic intervention in physical rehabilitation, the charge will be the same as similar therapy.

Q: Does insurance reimburse you for it?

A: Reimbursement is not an issue if the yoga therapy is done as a prescribed physical rehabilitative medicine procedure by a licensed rehab therapist. The therapist merely codes the procedures according to their therapeutic definition. Much of what is done in physical rehabilitation can be made "yogic" by transforming traditional interventions into mindful, embodied experiences for both patient and the therapist.

There are a few states and insurance companies that will allow billing for services directly by yoga teachers. Such a situation remains the exception and patients are best directed to check with their individual insurance carrier.

Suggested Readings

Desikachar TKV. *The Heart of Yoga: Developing a Personal Practice*. Rochester, VT: Inner Traditions; 1995.

Kraftsow G. *Yoga for Wellness: Healing with the Timeless Teachings of Viniyoga*. New York, NY: Penguin Compass; NY.

Yoga Alliance. Available at: http://www.yogaalliance.org

Yoga Biomedical Trust. Available at: http://www.yogatherapy.org

Yoga Research and Education Center. Available at: http://www.yrec.org

14

Spirituality and Health

Marilyn J. Schlitz, PhD

About the Author

Marilyn J. Schlitz is vice president for Research and Education at the Institute of Noetic Sciences and senior scientist at California Pacific Medical Center. Dr. Schlitz has conducted many studies addressing the role of intention on healing including a National Institutes of Health funded clinical trial on expectancy effects of distant healing for wound healing among women undergoing reconstructive surgery. She is a medical anthropologist and has a special interest in understanding the barriers to integration of consciousness-related approaches to health and healing and in the need for renewal and transformation for health professionals.

Q: What got you interested in working with spirituality?

A: My work over the past two decades involves the scientific and anthropological study of intention in healing, focusing primarily on distant healing as the focus of both field and laboratory based studies. This work speaks to a largely unexplored area that lies at the interface of consciousness and the physical world. This study area brings me directly into the world of spirituality; I have had the opportunity to work closely with spiritual teachers and practitioners from many traditions. In the process, I have come to view science as a spiritual practice that allows for a deep engagement with the mystery of life.

Q: What are the noetic sciences?

A: The field of noetic sciences investigates consciousness (mind and spirit) and the relationship of consciousness to the physical world. The Institute of Noetic Sciences (IONS) is the leading center for this exploration, using frontier sciences, transformative education, and learning communities to understand the expanded scope of human possibilities. The Institute of Noetic Science is an international nonprofit organization with 35,000 members and 280 self-organizing community groups throughout the world. It was founded in 1973 by Apollo 14 Astronaut Edgar Mitchell. I have been with IONS since 1994 and I currently hold the title of Vice President for Research and Education. In this capacity, I have the unique opportunity to learn about people's direct experiences with spirituality, to conduct research that allows us a deeper understanding of these experiences, and to create educational programs that help facilitate the application of our findings into daily life. This is often done with distant healing intentions (DHI), meaning there may be a physical separation from a few feet to thousands of miles between the healer and the recipient of the healing activity.

Distant healing intentions encompasses a broad range of healing practices, many of which are based in ancient spiritual traditions. Virtually all major religions, including Buddhism, Christianity, Islam, and Hinduism, endorse and encourage the use of distant healing among their adherents. Two of the most common distant healing practices are offering prayers for those who are ill and using forms of meditation where the practitioner holds a compassionate intention to relieve the suffering of another. Some practices focus on curing a very specific disease state while others emphasize creating a compassionate environment that can have a healing effect. Virtually all distant healing practices are concerned with alleviating the suffering and increasing the well being of others. Specific details of DHI and other modalities are available on the IONS website at **www.noetic.org**.

Q: How does spirituality factor in with the study of consciousness?

A: Consciousness is that aspect of ourselves that we experience most directly. It is the interior of our being: our subjective sense of self. Traditions that have looked most closely at consciousness, such as Buddhism, link an understanding of consciousness to the process of self-realization. Self, in this model, is not defined by the physical body, but involves a fundamental unity of all consciousness. In this sense, consciousness and spirituality are co-joined. In the Western technologically-based culture we live in, the focus is largely on the outer dimensions of reality. Consciousness has largely been ignored in any way other than as an epiphenomenon of the brain. Today, with the development of advanced brain imaging technology, combined with the proliferation of Eastern practices in the West, scientists have begun to take a fresh look at consciousness. In some cases, this means that scientists have begun to look at the Eastern practices not only as the focus of scientific inquiry, but also as a path of life that moves their work from an exclusive focus on the outer world to a deep reverence for the inner world of consciousness. In this process, a new form of spirituality is being born, one in which the researchers themselves are being transformed.

Q: What about cross cultural healing?

A: Health and healing have been basic human concerns throughout history and in every recorded culture. The understanding of what healing means, how it is achieved, and who can facilitate healing differs from culture to culture. Definitions of the body, for example, extend from the physical to multiple dimensions into subtle realms beyond the physical body. With such a range of approaches, it is easy to see how different views of health and well being have developed across cultures and throughout history.

Q: What is distant healing intention? How is it affected by spirituality and healing?

A: Distant healing encompasses a broad range of healing practices, many of which are based in ancient spiritual traditions. Virtually all major religions, including Buddhism, Christianity, Islam, and Hinduism, endorse and encourage the use of distant healing among their adherents. In a medical context, distant healing intention postulates that the intentions of one person can influence the health of a distant person.[1] In more general terms, DHI postulates that the intentions of one or more persons can interact with the physiological, psychological, and behavioral status of one or more distant living systems. DHI is a subset of a broader class of controversial phenomena suggesting the existence of direct mind-matter interactions.

Many terms are used to describe forms of distant healing interventions. They include intercessory prayer, spiritual healing, non-directed prayer, intentionality, energy healing, pranic healing, non-local healing, non-contact Therapeutic Touch, level III Reiki, external Qi Gong, and Johrei. Each of these terms describes a particular theoretical, cultural, and pragmatic approach to influencing a healing or biological change through mental intention of one person toward another.[2]

Q: How does distant healing work?

A: Different approaches to distant healing are rooted in very different worldviews and cosmologies and consequently there are numerous perspectives on how distant healing works. Common to virtually all perspectives is the belief that a person's focused intention can have a non-local effect, that is, the healing intention of one person can have a positive effect on another at a distance.

Specific explanations of how the healing effect occurs are based largely on the worldview of the healer. Some healers hold worldviews where God can intervene in a powerful way to alter physical reality, in which case it is God's action that brings about healing. Other healers hold worldviews where all reality is understood as being intimately interconnected and where mind and consciousness can have non-local effects. For these healers, it is the power of mind or consciousness itself that brings about a healing effect through the non-local transfer of either energy or information.

The idea that mental intention can causally influence distant living systems evokes two scientific problems:

1. "action at a distance" is impossible. Restated, this assumption presumes that all observable phenomena are causally connected, and that all causal connections must be proximally (i.e., spatiotemporally) contiguous. Thus a phenomenon based on "distant influence," with no known observable causal connections, is scientifically forbidden.
2. There are no accepted theoretical reasons to expect that mind can directly interact with matter, excepting perhaps a mind interacting with "its" brain.

These two problems are sufficient to cause most scientists to seriously doubt that DHI is genuinely "distant healing." As a result, it is understandable why skeptics assume that apparent DHI effects can be completely explained as a combination of wishful thinking, poor methodologies, embellishment, and in extreme cases, fraud. While thoroughly reviewing the theoretical implications of DHI is beyond the scope of this chapter, it is useful to point out that both of the above scientific objections to DHI have been obsolete for over a century. While Einstein complained about "spooky actions at a distance" in quantum mechanics, subsequent experiments have demonstrated that the fabric of the universe is indeed non-local, that is, it not only allows action at a distance but, the argument can be made, its very essence is non-local.[3–6] Likewise, the role of observation and consciousness in the physical world has been seriously discussed by virtually all of the founders of quantum theory,[7,8] suggesting that at some level mind and matter may be fundamentally inseparable.

Thus, while classical physics and "common sense" disallow the possibility of DHI phenomena, our most accurate theoretical descriptions of the physical world, as captured in the formalisms of modern physics, do provide an accepted physical substrate for DHI.

Q: **Can distant healing be taught or learned?**

A: There are various perspectives on the definition of a distant healer and how they should be trained. At the broadest level, many religious traditions maintain that anyone can be a distant healer and all that is required is a compassionate heart. In this sense, anyone who prays for healing for another is a distant healing practitioner. At the other end of the spectrum, some traditions believe that only certain people have the "gift" of healing, that this capacity is bestowed by the divine or God and is not available to all. A more nuanced perspective is that most people have healing capacities, but that training and practice is required to fully develop these capacities.

Researchers have observed that the quality most commonly held among distant healing practitioners is "an ability to hold a compassionate intention for another at a distance." From this perspective, distant healing can be understood as an "integral practice" that brings together a healer's capacities for holding intention, attention and compassion in ways that may enhance healing effects. Different traditions offer a variety of forms of training that can increase an individual's capability to hold intention and attention and express compassion, with some focusing more on the power of intention and attention and others on the effect of compassion. Some traditions, particularly those with a shamanic orientation, may require the healer to pass certain initiation rites and learn complex healing rituals.

Q: **Why do you believe in this?**

A: At a personal level, I believe spirituality provides a meaning system that makes life fuller and more purposeful. At a scientific level, there are many important research questions that still need to be addressed. Are there physical and psychological benefits of spiritual practice? What are the best ways to measure spirituality and its potential benefits? As a scientist, belief is not really the operative term. I think that there are enough reported benefits to justify taking spirituality, distant healing, and other alternative modalities seriously in terms of research and open-minded inquiry.

Q: **Does prayer and spirituality as a complementary and alternative practice really work?**

A: People commonly report positive outcomes related to DHI. As such, it is appropriate to ask what is happening. Is it due to suggestion, wishful thinking, or some complex placebo response? Or is there the possibility that thoughts are potent and that they can create changes in the physical world, even at a distance.

Q: How does it work?

A: To date, there are no explanations about the how and why of spiritual healing. Answers are based significantly on the assumptions that form the questions we ask. Is reality solely limited to the physical dimensions or are there aspects of reality that transcend the physical? Or is it some combination of the two?

Q: Where do I go for distant healing? And how do I find an alternative therapies practitioner?

A: There is currently a wider acceptance of distant healing within the spiritual and religious circles than within the medical and mental health community. The majority of distant healing practitioners have been trained and continue to work within the context of a specific spiritual tradition. Consequently, if you are comfortable with a particular spiritual tradition, that is often the best place to start your search. If you begin your search within a spiritual tradition, you should be aware of a few issues.

1. The term "distant healing" is used in research circles, but is often not used within religious or spiritual groups. In making inquiries you may want to use terminology more appropriate to your tradition such as "praying for healing of someone at a distance" or "meditation approaches where the focus is having compassion for one who is suffering."

2. Most healers employ a broad range of practices of which distant healing is only one, and there are few healers who focus solely on distant healing. You may have greater success seeking out individuals who refer to themselves as healers and then ask about their distant healing practices rather than looking strictly for distant healers.

3. Be persistent. Within most spiritual traditions there will be a range of attitudes regarding the efficacy of distant healing. Just because the first teacher or minister you speak with may not feel comfortable with or know of any distant healers, virtually all traditions have large constituencies who do believe in distant healing.

4. If you don't wish to be involved with a spiritual tradition but are interested in finding a distant healer, a good place to start is hospitals that have Complementary and Alternative Medicine (CAM) practices.

There are a growing number of physicians as well as other health practitioners such as chiropractors and psychotherapists who integrate CAM, integrative medicine, or holistic medicine approaches into their work. These health practitioners are often open to distant healing approaches and may be able to provide you with referrals. Another excellent resource in this area is the National Center for Complementary and Alternative Medicine, a program of the National Institutes of Health. Its website, available at

http://nccam.nih.gov, offers a very helpful set of guidelines for exploring alternative approaches to health and healing.

A primary commitment of The Institute of Noetic Sciences is conducting independent research in areas of health and healing and, consequently, it does not make recommendations or endorse individual health practitioners or particular approaches to healing.

Q: What is the difference between healing and curing?

A: Two of the most common distant healing practices are offering prayers for those who are ill and using forms of meditation where the practitioner holds a compassionate intention to relieve the suffering of another. Some practices focus on curing a very specific disease state while others emphasize creating a compassionate environment that can have a healing effect. Virtually all distant healing practices are concerned with alleviating the suffering and increasing the well being of others.

Q: Can the mind, consciousness, and spirit help the body heal?

A: Healing can be facilitated through social support, lifestyle choices, psychological well being and a greater feeling of purpose. How these translate to physical changes is still to be determined.

Q: Is the study of consciousness part of a religious movement or cult?

A: Science offers a system of rigor and discernment that allows us to approach to consciousness from the perspective of open-minded inquiry. This provides a good opportunity to challenge our assumptions and gain a new depth of understanding about ourselves and our place in the Universe.

Q: I have experienced psi phenomena, such as telepathy or precognition. What can I do about it?

A: The vast majority of people report having some kind of psi or extrasensory experience. There are many books written on this topic, most grounded in personal experiences, some focusing on the evidence for psi from a scientific perspective. A useful book on this topic, called *The Conscious Universe*, was written by my colleague, Dr. Dean Radin.[9] The IONS website also offers a series of online games that allow people to experiment with their own abilities. These are available at **www.noetic.org** and are called the Garden of Dreams.

Q: Can psi abilities be misused?

A: It is my perspective that anything that can be used for good can be used for bad. Larry Dossey has written a helpful book on this called *Be Careful What You Pray For . . . You Just Might Get It.*[10]

Q: How many people believe in this practice?

A: It is difficult to quantify the prevalence of the use of DHI as a complementary and alternative medicine therapy in the United States because it is so commonly practiced within American religious and spiritual life. The following studies may give you an idea of the prevalence.

- 82% of Americans believe in the healing power of prayer; 64% of Americans feel that physicians should pray with patients who request it.[11]
- 19% of cancer patients report they have augmented their conventional medical care with prayer or spiritual healing.[12]
- 88% of women in the American Cancer Society's support groups for women with breast cancer found spiritual or religious practice important in coping with their illness,[13] although the extent to which specific prayers or intentions of healing were part of their activities was not clear.
- 96% of patients stated that they prayed for their health before going in for surgery.[14]
- In certain cultural or ethnic groups, seeking healing prayers or spiritual healing from an identified practitioner is commonplace.[15]

As a whole, the population of the United Kingdom is less traditionally religious than the United States, but there are more distant healers in the United Kingdom (approximately 14,000) than there are therapists from any other branch of CAM.[16] This indicates that DHI is widely practiced independently of religious backgrounds.

Spiritual healing, energy healing, and prayer are rapidly gaining acceptance among conventional medical professionals.

- In a 1996 survey of Northern California physicians,[11] 13% reported using or recommending prayer or religious healing as an intervention.
- Non-Contact Therapeutic Touch is used formally by nurses in at least 80 hospitals within the United States,[17] and has been taught to more that 43,000 healthcare professionals.[18]
- Among the lay public, Reiki International, one of the largest training organizations for "subtle-energy healing" therapies, reports having certified more than 500,000 practitioners worldwide. While Reiki healing is frequently performed through physical contact, one form of Reiki is claimed to be effective over distances of thousands of miles.[19] For more information see Chapter 20 on Reiki.

Q: What type of research has been done?

A: Despite only modest scientific proof of its efficacy and a lack of adequate theoretical explanations, many people regularly use some form of DHI, such as prayer, in the hope that it will help friends and loved ones who are ill. The problem is that in addition to doubt about its efficacy, even those who regularly practice DHI don't know how much, how often, or how long they should practice DHI to be effective. These are the types of questions addressed by both clinical and laboratory DHI research.

Anecdotal claims of DHI have been reported in a wide variety of conditions ranging from malignancies and genetic illnesses to wounds.[20] In a narrative review of controlled experimental and clinical studies published before 2001, Benor[21,22] found statistically significant evidence for such effects. The extent of selective reporting in that literature is unknown, and many of those studies did not use double-blind, randomized trial designs.[21,22]

In addition, several randomized, double-blind investigations support the clinical efficacy of DHI.[16,23,24] Based on a systematic review that was recently published in the *Annals of Internal Medicine*,[16] Astin et al. reported that approximately 57% of the randomized, controlled trials reviewed showed a positive treatment effect in a wide range of human populations.

Q: How much does it cost?

A: Compassionate intention or DHI is one of the least costly forms of CAM; in many cases, it is practiced free of charge.

Q: Are there any consequences to your health?

A: Thus far, the data suggests that religious and spiritual practice is beneficial to one's health.[20] There are also a series of basic science and clinically based experiments that suggest that DHI also has therapeutic benefit.[16] Clearly more data need to be collected to better understand issues related to dose, distance, as well as a range of psychosocial variables that may or may not be important.

Q: What will my doctor think of this?

A: More and more, members of the medical community are opening to the beliefs and practices of their patients. The best advice is to choose a practitioner with whom one feels trust and confidence in their abilities to help the patient heal. If this requires that the physician maintain a similar belief system, this can be one of the questions one asks when choosing a provider.

Q: Do I need to approve it with my doctor before I start using it?

A: Not at all, although it is always helpful to share as much information with your health provider as possible.

Q: Are you certified or licensed in what you do?

A: I am trained in research and am not a healthcare provider.

Q: How long did you go to school to do this?

A: The time it takes to complete graduate school. In my case, this was a nine year process, plus an additional two years of post doctoral study.

Q: Where can I read more about this?

A: The most extensive place for reliable information on DHI or compassionate intention is the IONS website available at **www.noetic.org**.

Q: What might be different in the world if everyone believed they had some ability to heal themselves and others?

A: As we find ourselves in a relational universe, connected rather than disconnected from others, we become more responsible for ourselves and others in ways that bring about greater compassion, altruism, and gratefulness. This can only help us as we seek to heal the planet.

References

1. Schlitz M, Radin DI, Malle BF, Schmidt S, Utts J, Yount GL. Distant healing intention: Definitions and evolving guidelines for laboratory studies. *Altern Ther Health Med.* 2003;9(3):A31–A43.

2. Schlitz M, Braud W. Distant intentionality and healing: assessing the evidence. *Altern Ther Health Med.* 1997;3(6):62–73.

3. Accardi L, Regoli M. Non-locality and quantum theory: new experimental evidence. Accessed December 22, 2005. http://volterra.mat.uniroma2.it.

4. Kwiat PG, Barraza-Lopez S, Stefanov A. Gisin N. Experimental entanglement distillation and "hidden" non-locality. *Nature.* 2001:409:1014–1017.

5. Namiki M. Some controversies in the epistemology of modern physics. In: Luhmann N, Maturana HR, Namiki M, Redder V, Varela FJ, eds. *Beobachter: Konvergenz der Erkenntnistheorie* München: Fink; 1990:25–46.

6. Rowe, MA, Kielpinski D, Meyer V, Sackett CA, Itano WM, Monroe C, Wineland DJ. Experimental violation of a Bell's inequality with efficient detection. *Nature.* 2001;409:791–794.

7. Stapp HP. Quantum theory and the physicist's conception of nature: Philosophical implications of Bell's theorem. In: Kitchener RF, ed. *The World View of Contemporary Physics: Does It Need a New Metaphysics?* Albany, NY: State University of New York Press; 1988:38–58.

8. Stapp HP. The Copenhagen interpretation. *J Mind Behavior.* 1997;18:127–154.

9. Radin DI. *The Conscious Universe: The Scientific Truth of Psychic Phenomena.* San Francisco, CA: Harper Collins; 1997.

10. Dossey L. (1997). *Be Careful What You Pray For . . . You Just Might Get It.* New York: Harper Collins.

11. Wallis C. Faith and healing. *Time.* 1996;147(26):58–64.

12. Cassileth BR. Contemporary unorthodox treatment in cancer medicine. *Ann Intern Med,* 1984;101:105–112.

13. Johnson SC, Spilka B. Coping with breast cancer: the roles of clergy and faith. *J Relig Health.* 1991;20:21–33.

14. Saudia TL, Kinney MR, et al. Health locus of control and helpfulness of prayer. *Heart Lung.* 1991;20(1):60–65.

15. Suarez M, Raffaelli M, O'leary A. Use of folk healing practices by HIV-infected Hispanics living in the United States. *AIDS Care.* 1996;8(6):683–690.

16. Astin JA, Harkness E, Ernst E. The efficacy of "distant healing": a systematic review of randomized trials. *Ann Intern Med* 2000;132(11):903–910.

17. Maxwell J. Nursing's new age? *Christianity Today.* 1996;40(3)96–99.

18. Krieger D. *The Therapeutic Touch: How to Use Your Hands to Help or Heal.* Englewood Cliffs, NJ, Prentice-Hall; 1979.

19. Schlitz M, Braud W. Reiki plus natural healing: an ethnographic and experimental study. *Psi Research.* 1985;4:100–123.

20. Dossey L. *Healing Words: The Power of Prayer and the Practice of Medicine.* San Francisco, CA: Harper; 1993.

21. Benor DJ. *Spiritual Healing: Scientific Validation of a Healing Revolution.* Southfield, MI: Vision; 2001.

22. Benor DJ. *Spiritual Healing: Scientific Validation of a Healing Revolution. Professional Supplement.* Southfield, MI: Vision; 2002.

23. Roberts L, Ahmed I, Hall S. Intercessory prayer for the alleviation of ill health. *Cochrane Database Syst Rev.* 2000;(2):CD000368.

24. Schlitz M, Lewis N. The healing powers of prayer. *Noetic Sci Rev.* 1996;Summer: 29–33.

15

Herbal Medicines and Other Natural Products

Patrick Miederhoff, PhD, PharmD

About the Author

Patrick Miederhoff is a retired professor of pharmacy from Virginia Commonwealth University in Richmond. He currently serves as director of Alternative Medicine for a large primary care organization, PatientFirst. He continues to do research in alternative medicine and provides lectures on the topic to professional and lay groups.

Q: How long have you been interested in herbal medicine?

A: When I was in pharmacy school in the early 1960s, I had to take course-work in an area called pharmacognosy. Pharmacognospy is the science of drugs derived from natural sources. This was my first exposure to herbs and I was fascinated then and have been ever since.

Q: What are herbal medicines and natural products?

A: "Natural products" is a term applied to any medicine that has a natural ori-gin. They could be from plants, animals, or other natural sources. Examples would be things like thyroid hormone from pigs, ginger root, beneficial bacteria like *Lactobacillus acidophilus*, glucosamine, melatonin, and leaves from the gingko tree. All of these substances tend to be lumped into herbal medicines, but technically only plant-derived medicines are called herbals. Herbs can be made from the whole plant or from the specific parts like leaves, barks, roots, or flowers.

Q: How are herbal medicines prepared?

A: The plant or plant parts are harvested and then dried. Sometimes the dried plant material is used as a medicine, for example, chewing ginseng root or making a tea from sassafras bark. However, usually an extract is made from the dried plant material using various solvents such as water or alcohol. Traditional herbalists feel strongly about making their own products because they want them to be minimally processed. I recommend using commercially made standardized products for safety and other reasons.

Standardization refers to adjusting the amount of active constituents in an herbal preparation to provide uniformity of active constituents across batches. This process helps to insure consistent effectiveness of the product. For example, St. John's wort is usually standardized to contain 0.3% hyper-icum. Traditional herbalists object to standardization because it involves further processing of the herbal material.

Q: How do natural products differ from pharmaceuticals?

A: Pharmaceuticals:
  • have distinct chemical entities,
  • go through rigorous testing,
  • are approved by the US Food and Drug Administration (FDA),
  • are used for prevention and treatment of disease,
  • are more powerful medicines, and
  • have unwanted toxic effects.
    Natural products:
  • have not usually been studied extensively,
  • are not approved by the FDA for treatment of disease,
  • are milder, and
  • have less unwanted toxic effects.

Q: How do herbal medicines work?

A: Because herbs have not been extensively studied, we frequently do not know how they work from a pharmacological point of view. We assume that some chemical constituent in the herb interacts with the chemistry of the body to bring about some positive change but we usually do not understand it. In some instances, certain herbs have been used for thousands of years with success, so we do not feel compelled to understand how they work. It would be very costly to research these products when they are being used with safe and effective outcomes.

What little research that is being done is following a pharmacological paradigm, looking for a mechanism of action that may be similar to synthetic pharmacological agents. For example, the herb valerian is thought to produce sedative effects by influencing gamma-amino butyric acid (GABA) neurotransmitters.[1,2] This happens to be the same mechanism by which the benzodiazepines class of drugs works. However, the familiarality of the names Valium® and valerian is purely coincidental, even though it is believed that these medicines work by similar means and produce similar effects.

Q: How widespread is the use of herbal medicine?

A: The most frequently used modality in complementary and alternative practices and products is herbal medicine. Surveys indicate that approximately 50% of all adults in the United States have used some form of natural products.

Q: What are the most commonly used herbs?

A: The United States use of herbal medicine is influenced by European herbal medicine. In recent years, we have seen increasing use of herbs from Asia, especially Indian and China. Examples of this would be tumeric, a good anti-inflammatory agent, from India and astragalus for immune support from China. Top selling herbs in the United States are seen in **Table 15.1**.

Table 15.1   Top Selling Herbs in the United States

Gingko	For age-related memory loss, senility, dementia
Ginseng	For energy and stress
Garlic	For lowering cholesterol and an anti-infective
Echinacea	For immune support
Saw palmetto	For prostate problems
Soy	For a source of quality protein and hormone balance
Kava	For anxiety
Cranberry	For bladder infections
Flax	As a source of fiber and other important nturients
Valerian	For a sleep aid
Black cohosh	For symptoms of menopause
Milk thistle	For liver support

Q: Are herbal medicines safe to use? What are the risks involved when using herbs?

A: As said earlier, the FDA does not approve herbal medicines for the treatment of disease. Herbal medicines are allowed on the market as dietary supplements. They do not have to be proven effective, but the FDA monitors their safety. An example is the current concern for the safety of ephedra and kava that were recently taken off the market by the FDA.

In general, herbs are safe when used as recommended, but they are not risk free. The consumer needs to take some responsibility for gaining some basic understanding of herbal medicine and to have confidence in any practitioner they may consult.

Herbal medicines are safer than conventional medicines because they are more dilute and less likely to be toxic, but caution is still important. Harvesting wild herbs is not advised because of the possibility of misidentification and contamination with herbicides. Herb use during pregnancy is not advised even though ginger is widely used to treat morning sickness. The safety of ginger for this purpose comes from long-term and widespread use without any apparent teratogenic effects.

Q: Are there studies showing herbal medicines to be effective?

A: European countries make more use of herbal medicine than the United States, consequently, most of the studies on effectiveness have been done in Europe. Many health professionals in the United States are under the impression that there is little or no research in this area. While there is not the level of research as there is on pharmaceuticals, some studies do exist. Also, because of the widespread use in the United States, the National Institutes of Health is beginning to sponsor studies on natural products as well as other alternative medications.

Q: How do herbal medicines compare in cost to pharmaceuticals?

A: For a pharmaceutical to be approved by the FDA, there has to be considerable research in place on safety and effectiveness. This can be an expensive process, costing as much as $500 million dollars for one drug to get through the approval process. This dramatically increases the cost of pharmaceuticals making them more expensive than herbal medicines. Since herbal medicines do not have to go through this process, the cost to purchase herbs is much less.

Q: How does a consumer know which product to buy?

A: One of the problems in the herbal market is the chaos related to the quality of the product and indication for use. The Dietary Supplement Health Education Act of 1994 included a definition of a dietary supplement which included herbals, botanicals, and other products derived from plant materials. This was the first attempt to regulate these products by the government. It was also mandated that indications on the use of herbs and natural products could not be put on the product label because there is lack of research to support this implication. This may have confused consumers even more as to what to buy and for what.

Problems still exists. There is little constraint on what products can be used in health promotion or disease prevention. There is no clear cut policy on reporting adverse events from herbs and natural products. And there is little quality control that regulates the standardization of products. To assist the consumer in purchasing products, there is now a website, **www.consumerlab.com**, that evaluates natural products. ConsumerLab.com, LLC, is a privately owned company and is not affiliated with manufacturers of health and nutrition products. For a small fee, a consumer can subscribe and get reliable information on a product that has been tested, results and information are provided to help consumers and healthcare professionals evaluate health, wellness, and nutrition products.

Q: **If my doctor prescribes an herbal product, will it be paid for by my health insurance company?**

A: Not likely! Herbal products are not generally included in the formularies of health insurers. However, things are starting to change in this area. Some insurers are starting to cover alternative therapies and hopefully this will include herbal medicines.

Q: **What do medical doctors think about herbal medicines?**

A: Unfortunately, most regard this area as quackery. This is unfortunate because this attitude makes it difficult for patients to talk to their doctors about their use of natural products. This also is beginning to change. More doctors are becoming knowledgeable and are able to provide guidance to patients in this area. The Institute of Medicine (IOM) convened a study committee to explore scientific, policy, and practice questions that arise from the significant and increasing use of Complementary and Alternative Medicine (CAM) therapies by the American public. In the report "Use of Complementary and Alternative Medicine (CAM) by the American Public" it was recommended to amend the regulation of supplements to improve quality control and consumer protections and to create incentives for research on the efficacy of these products.[3]

Q: **Does a person need to be concerned about drugs interacting with herbs?**

A: Definitely! There is beginning to be some documentation on how drugs and herbs interact. Pharmacists tend to be the best informed in this area and can provide guidance to help avoid potential interactions. Some examples of interactions are listed here.

- Dong quai increases the anticoagulant effect of warfarin.[4,5]
- St. John's Wort decreases the effectiveness of digoxin.[6]
- Kava increases the sedative effects of alprazolam.[7]
- Ephedra, caffeine, and stimulants may raise blood pressure.[8]
- Melatonin will cause increased sedation with antidepressants and hormones.[9,10]
- Valerian will cause excessive drowsiness when used with other sedatives.[11]
- Alpha lipoic acid may increase the effectiveness of diabetic medications; insulin and oral anti-diabetic medications may need to be decreased.[12]

For more drug interactions with herbs, the following web pages may be helpful in finding more information: **http://www.rdgp.com.au/pharm** and **http://www.drugdigest.org/DD/Interaction/ChooseDrugs**.

Q: What professional credentials should I look for when consulting with someone about herbal medicines?

A: There is no formal credentialing process for herbalists in the United States. The American Herbalist Guild (AHG) has professional membership so anyone with AHG after their name has demonstrated competence as an herbalist. Naturopathic physicians that have graduated from an accredited naturopathic medical school are very well trained in herbal medicine. A medical doctor that is a member of a professional organization like the American Holistic Medical Association is usually knowledgeable in herbal medicine. Some pharmacies specialize in natural products and provide both reliable products and guidance.

There is a specialty within botany known as pharmacognosy that was mentioned earlier. This is the science of identifying useful drugs from plant sources. These scientists are usually working in universities and other agencies rather than working as practitioners in herbal medicine. The one exception is James Duke, PhD, who has written extensively for the lay public on herbal medicine (see Suggested Readings).

Several formal training programs exist in the United States. Bastyr University (**http://www.bastyr.edu**) in Seattle has an undergraduate degree program in herbal sciences. The Tai Sophia Institute in Laurel, Maryland, (**http://tai.vmtllc.com**) has a master's degree program in botanical healing. It should be noted that the term "master herbalist" does not mean that the practitioner has a masters degree in herbal medicine.

Q: What do you see for the future of herbal medicine?

A: We have to recognize that the whole movement toward natural approaches to health is one of consumer preference. This is a grass roots movement that will not go away and cannot be stopped. With wider acceptance on the part of the healthcare system, we will see a continued growth in all areas of natural medicine, including herbal medicine.

Currently, disease treatment claims cannot be made for herbal medicines since that prerogative is limited to FDA approved drugs in the United States. Because of the increasing popularity of natural medicine, it is likely that herbal medicines will make gains toward greater legal privilege. For example, if research demonstrates that an herb is effective for a particular disease indication, the FDA may be forced to allow disease treatment claims be made by herbal companies and practitioners.

Suggested Readings

Duke J. *The Green Pharmacy: The Ultimate Compendium of Natural Remedies From The World's Foremost Authority On Healing Herbs (Green Pharmacy)*. New York, NY: Rodale Press Inc.;1997.

Facts and Comparisons. *Guide to Popular Natural Products*. 3rd ed. Philadelphia, PA: Lippincott & Williams; 2003.

Hoffman D. *The Herbal Handbook: A User's Guide to Medical Herbalism*. Rochester, VT: Healing Arts Press; 1998.

Murray M, Pizzomo J. *Encyclopedia of Natural Medicine*. 2nd ed. Roseville, CA: Prima Publishing; 1998.

Natural Medicines Comprehensive Database. Available at: www.naturaldatabase.com

AltMedDex® System. Available at: www.micromeddex.com/products/altmedex/

References

1. Glass JR, Sproule BA, Herrmann N, Streiner D, Busto UE. Acute pharmacological effects of temazepam, diphenhydramine, and valerian in healthy elderly subjects. *J Clin Psychopharmacol,* 2003;23(3):260–268.

2. Houghton, PJ. The scientific basis for the reputed activity of Valerian. *J Pharm Pharmacol.* 1999;51(5):505–512.

3. Institute of Medicine. Use of Complementary and Alternative Medicine (CAM) by the American public. Available at: http://www.iom.edu/?id=4829&redirect=0. Accessed December 23, 2005. 12. Lee WJ, Song KH, Koh EH, Won JC, Kim HS, Park HS, Kim MS, Kim SW, Lee KU, Park JY. Alpha-lipoic acid increases insulin sensitivity by activating AMPK in skeletal muscle. *Biochem Biophys Res Commun.* 2005;332(3):885–891.

4. Heck AM, DeWitt BA, Lukes AL. Potential interactions between alternative therapies and warfarin. *Am J Health Syst Pharm.* 2000;57(13):1221–1227.

5. Page RL, Lawrence JD. Potentiation of warfarin by dong quai. *Pharmacotherapy.* 1999;19(7):870–876.

6. Mueller SC, Uehleke B, Woehling H, Petzsch M, Majcher-Peszynska J, Hehl EM, Sievers H, Frank B, Riethling AK, Drewelow B. Effect of St John's wort dose and preparations on the pharmacokinetics of digoxin. *Clin Pharmacol Ther.* 2004; 75(6):546–557.

7. Almeida JC, Grimsley EW. Coma from the health food store: interaction between kava and alprazolam. *Ann Intern Med.* 1996;125(11):940–941.

8. Vukovich MD, Schoorman R, Heilman C, Jacob P, Benowitz NL. Caffeine-herbal ephedra combination increases resting energy expenditure, heart rate and blood pressure. *Clin Exp Pharmacol Physiol.* 2005;32(1–2):47–53.

9. Golombek DA, Pevet P, Cardinali DP. Melatonin effects on behavior: possible mediation by the central GABAergic system. *Neurosci Biobehav Rev.* 1996;20(3): 403–412.

10. Wong PT, Ong YP. Acute antidepressant-like and antianxiety-like effects of tryptophan in mice. *Pharmacol.* 2001:62(3):151–156.

11. Ugalde M, Reza V, Gonzalez-Trujano ME, Avula B, Khan IA, Navarrete A. Isobolographic analysis of the sedative interaction between six central nervous system depressant drugs and Valeriana edulis hydroalcoholic extract in mice. *J Pharm Pharmacol.* 2005;57(5):631–639.

16

Chiropractic Medicine

Dana J. Lawrence, FICC, DC

About the Author

Dana J. Lawrence is an associate professor at the Palmer Center for Chiropractic Research at Palmer College of Chiropractic. He was formerly the dean of the Lincoln College of Postprofessional, Graduate and Continuing Education; director of the Department of Publication and Editorial Review; and professor of the Department of Chiropractic Practice at the National University of Health Sciences. He is editor emeritus of the *Journal of Manipulative and Physiological Therapeutics* (the sole journal in the chiropractic profession to be indexed in Index Medicus and Current Contents/Clinical Medicine, along with other international databases), and past editor for other journals. He has published a number of textbooks. He was a member of the Ad Hoc Committee for the Office of Alternative Medicine, and later became a member of the Alternative Medicine Program Advisory Council of the National Institute of Health Office of Alternative Medicine and the National Center for Complementary and Alternative Medicine.

Q: What got you interested in chiropractic medicine?

A: I wish that I had a dramatic story to tell you, but the truth is that I fell into chiropractic by accident. I had graduated from Michigan State University with a degree in biology and a minor in botany, and was considering careers in one of three disciplines: healthcare, high-energy physics, or humanities. After returning to Michigan State for a further course of study in medical technology, I applied for masters programs in biology at Wayne State, Oakland University, and University of Detroit and was accepted by them all. But a chance meeting with my father, long divorced from my mother, led to him giving me a copy of a catalog from the National College of Chiropractic; he had been working on a radio ad for a local chiropractor. I applied to National knowing little about chiropractic, but was soon accepted. Once there, I became more and more interested in chiropractic. This led to a position at the college once I graduated, and the rest, as they say, is history.

Q: Why do you believe in chiropractic medicine?

A: It is not a matter of belief. It is a matter of combining the evidence with clinical experience and academic study. There is ample evidence supporting the use of chiropractic manipulation in a variety of conditions, and for many others, the care rendered is similar to that from any other healthcare practitioner.

Q: Does chiropractic medicine really work?

A: Yes, and no. One can't really speak of whether chiropractic works. The better question to ask is, when does it work? For what kinds of problems will chiropractic intervention confer a benefit? For that, we turn to research and find that there are numerous conditions which respond favorably to chiropractic care, chief and most well-known among them being low-back pain, neck pain, and headache. One important reference for information pertaining to the use of manipulation for low back pain is the clinical practice guidelines from the Agency for Health Care Policy and Research.[1] This summarizes research on the management of back pain.

Q: How many people use chiropractic medicine?

A: Studies from David Eisenberg have shown that approximately 12% of the American population uses chiropractic care.[2]

Q: How does it work?

A: In its most basic terms, chiropractic operates on the concept of *vis medicatrix naturae*; that is, the innate ability of the human body to heal itself. Chiropractors look to the nervous system as playing an important part in health and disease. When subluxation or joint dysfunction is present in the human body, it can interfere with the ability of the neuromusculoskeletal system to efficiently operate, and can lead to or contribute to the presence of disease. Thus, one of the major goals of chiropractic care is to locate and identify the nature of these subluxations, and to then treat them to eliminate them. This is done alongside standard medical diagnostic examination. Subluxation, in its most general definition, is a motion segment in which alignment, movement integrity, and physiologic function are altered though contacts between joint surfaces remain intact.[3]

Q: What are the principle concepts of chiropractic?

A: There are four principle concepts in chiropractic.

1. The nervous system influences all other body systems and plays an important role in maintaining health or in disease.
2. The human body has an innate ability to heal itself.
3. Subluxation interferes with the body's ability to maintain homeostasis and can contribute to the presence of illness.
4. It is necessary to diagnose and treat these subluxations.

Q: What kinds of conditions do you treat?

A: We are best known for our care of neuromusculoskeletal conditions, such as low-back pain, neck pain, and headache. However, chiropractors are primary-care providers and as such are responsible for the accurate diagnosis of most conditions that affect the human body. This includes organic conditions. An editorial I wrote in the *Journal of Manipulative Physiology Therapy* discusses case reports of chiropractic treatments indicating a breadth of experience in diagnosis and management.[4]

Q: Can manipulation help non-musculoskeletal conditions?

A: The information available here is less definitive. I should note that manipulation is only one form of treatment that chiropractic offers and forms only part of our approach to management. Even if manipulation may be of little-known benefit, there is still reason to seek chiropractic care for many conditions. However, certainly there is a substantial amount of research, and conditions such as hypertension, asthma, infantile colic, otitis media, gastric ulcer, and other conditions have received attention. A more complete survey of the research base for the management of organic conditions can be found in the textbook *Chiropractic Technique*.[5]

Q: How much does it cost?

A: Depending on the region, a general first office visit may run in the vicinity of $100 or more, though average office visits are less. Most insurance and managed-care providers cover chiropractic.

Q: Are there any consequences to my health? Is chiropractic dangerous?

A: Like most medical procedures, there is a small element of risk. Perhaps the most well known is the risk of cervical spinal cord damage or arterial dissection with cervical manipulation. Research from Paul Shekelle has estimated the risk of such damage as extremely small.[6] Chiropractic physicians are trained to perform appropriate tests prior to manipulation to rule out the possibility of such complications.

Q: What type of research has been done?

A: Way too much to present in any detail. The profession has published a peer-review and internationally indexed scientific journal, *The Journal of Manipulative and Physiological Therapeutics*, for 25 years now, which I currently edit. This, along with other biomedical journals within and without chiropractic, has helped present the state of our research. This research covers such general disciplines as basic science, clinical studies, health-services research, outcomes research, patient satisfaction studies, meta-analysis, qualitative research. and even historical and sociological research.

Q: How do I know it is working and not something else I am doing?

A: I am not sure how to answer this, since it seems to me that any practitioner could ask this question about any intervention.

Q: What will my doctor think about this? Do I need to approve it with my doctor before I start seeing a chiropractor?

A: If your medical doctor is aware of the strengths of chiropractic he or she should have no qualms or concerns whatsoever. Certainly you do not need the approval of a medical physician to see a chiropractor; chiropractors are licensed physicians in every state in the nation.

Q: Will this hurt me in the long run?

A: Simple answer: no.

Q: Does it interact with any medications I am taking?

A: Very likely not. However, it would be wise to inform your chiropractor of any medication you are taking, for this may indicate other conditions you may have and may help to ensure that treatments are appropriately used. An example of this is if you were taking medication for bone loss, this would be important for a chiropractor to know.

Q: Tell me about how you become a chiropractor. How long does it take to become a chiropractor? What is the course of study? What kinds of topics are you taught?

A: The course of study is five years in length with three main components to the curriculum: basic science, clinical science and clinical internship. See **Table 16.1** for a curriculum description.

Table 16.1   Curriculum for Chiropractic Medicine

Basic science	Anatomy, physiology, microbiology, histology and other areas	Earlier portions of training
Clinical science courses	Diagnostic classes like, cardio-vascular, neurology, orthopedics, radiology, general diagnosis, rehabilitation, nutrition, and others	Mid-portion of education prior to the internship
	Medical diagnosis with the more specific forms of chiropractic diagnosis and therapy, such as motion palpation, spinography and various forms of chiropractic technique	
Clinical internship	Final part of training	Patient care

In total, there is nearly 5000 hours of training. Today, the emphasis is upon problem-based education, similar to medical training. This is case-based, and integrates basic and clinical science far more than the more familiar didactic training with which we are all familiar. Assessment is also becoming important, with innovative assessment methods being used, including objective structured clinical examinations (OSCE exams) and the use of simulated patients where actual ones are not available.

Q: Are chiropractors certified or licensed?

A: Chiropractors are licensed and regulated similar to medical physicians in all 50 states and many countries around the world.[7]

Q: Can a chiropractor specialize?

A: Yes. Specialties include orthopedics, neurology, radiology, sports medicine, internal medicine, rehabilitation, and nutrition.

Q: Is chiropractic education accredited?

A: Yes. Our professional education program (programmatic accreditation) is accredited by the Commission on Accreditation of the Council on Chiropractic Education. We are also accredited by various local agencies. The National

University of Health Sciences is accredited by the North Central Association of Colleges and Schools, while other colleges receive their accreditation from their regional accrediting body (professional accreditation).

Q: Is continuing education required?

A: Yes. All states set requirements for continuing education, and this varies on a state-by-state basis.

Q: Who are some of the important people in chiropractic, both historically and currently?

A: A variety of people have contributed to chiropractic medicine. The works of these people have made chiropractic medicine what it is today. See **Table 16.2** for past contributors to chiropractic medicine.

Some of the current leaders in chiropractic medicine include those listed in **Table 16.3**. This is hardly a complete list and there are many, many other individuals who contribute daily to the overall health of the chiropractic profession. I do not mean to slight any by not noting them here.

Q: Is there anywhere I can read more about this? Web page information? Are there chiropractic journals? What about textbooks for chiropractors and chiropractic students?

A: Numerous books exist, but a wonderful text for the lay person is *Contemporary Chiropractic*, by Dr. Daniel Redwood.[8] Many other texts have been published and all are uniformly good. To learn more about chiropractic medicine, please see the recommended Suggested Readings at the end of this chapter.

Each chiropractic college maintains its own web site, and they can easily be found via a standard search engine such as **google.com**.

Numerous trade publications abound as well, such as *Dynamic Chiropractic*, *Journal of the American Chiropractic Association*, *International Chiropractic Association Journal*, and others.

Q: What are the future prospects for chiropractic?

A: The profession has undergone unprecedented growth over the past 15 years. There are now over 70,000 practicing chiropractors in the United States, making chiropractic the second largest general healthcare profession, behind medicine yet ahead of osteopathy. With the growth in high-quality rigorous research, coupled with innovative methodologies in chiropractic education institutions, the future looks very bright indeed.

Table 16.2   Past Contributors to Chiropractic Medicine

Daniel David Palmer (1845–1913)

- founder of the chiropractic profession
- a grocer and a magnetic healer, as well as a seeker after knowledge
- first chiropractic adjustment was by Palmer to Harvey Lillard
- founded the first school of chiropractic
- Palmer College of Chiropractic, now part of the Palmer University system, is still located today in Davenport, IA.

Bartlett Joshua Palmer (1882–1961)

- Palmer's son
- developer and promoter of chiropractic
- helped the profession grow and resist medical opposition

John Howard (1876–1954)

- founder of the National School of chiropractic, which later became the National College of Chiropractic and is today the National University of Health Sciences, the leading progressive chiropractic institution
- created what is known as the rational approach to chiropractic, based upon rigorous scientific training

Willard Carver (1866–1943)

- helped to codify a systems-based approach to subluxation
- believed that subluxation in the spine could lead to compensatory changes elsewhere in the spine
- influenced early legislative and regulatory efforts by the profession

John Nugent (1891–1971)

- altered the educational system in the profession
- made it possible for the profession's educational programs to receive both professional and programmatic accreditation
- helped to standardize the general chiropractic curriculum, and led to the demise of fly-by-night, mail order, and poorly managed chiropractic institutions
- helped chiropractic institutions become nonprofit and professionally owned

Joseph Janse (1909–1985)

- instrumental in helping to found the Council on Chiropractic Education, the National Board of Chiropractic Examiners, the Federation of Chiropractic Licensing Boards, the radiology residency program, scientific councils and the most influential scientific publication, the *Journal of Manipulative and Physiological Therapeutics*

Table 16.3   Current Contributors to Chiropractic Medicine

Scott Haldeman

- a chiropractor, PhD anatomist, and medical physician
- chiropractic researcher for the last two decades
- editor for a singularly influential text, *Modern Developments in the Principles and Practice of Chiropractic*[9]
- written extensively in the chiropractic and medical literature about the profession and has helped to bring its members into contact with researchers from other discipline areas

John Triano

- director for chiropractic services at the Texas Back Institute
- influential researcher within the profession for many years
- work, biomechanical in nature, has helped to define subluxation
- developed the functional spinal lesion model which is setting the agenda for future research

Louis Sportelli

- national spokesman for chiropractic
- incredibly influential is the political and legislative realm for chiropractic
- contributing to insurance equity and managed care topics
- works with the National Chiropractic Mutual Insurance Company

James Winterstein

- retiring president of the National University of Health Care
- vigilant efforts to move chiropractic further toward full primary-care rights and privileges
- developed the first full problem based learning (PBL) educational program, emphasizing primary care education

David Chapman-Smith

- attorney
- heads the World Federation of Chiropractic, which represents the interests of chiropractic organizations from many countries around the world

Suggested Readings

American Chiropractic Association. Available at: www.amerchiro.org

Foundation for Chiropractic Education and Research. Available at: www.fcer.org

World Federation of Chiropractic. Available at: www.wfc.org

Federation of Chiropractic Licensing Boards. Available at: www.fclb.org

Council on Chiropractic Education. Available at: www.cce-usa.org

Council of Chiropractic State Organizations. Available at: www.cocsa.org

International Chiropractic Association. Available at: www.chiropractic.org

Journal of Manipulative and Physiological Therapeutics. Available at:
www.mosby.com/jmpt

Journal of Chiropractic Medicine. Available at: www.journalchiromed.com

Chiropractic Journal of Australia. Available at: www.caa.com.au/cja/cjaindex.htm

Journal of the Canadian Chiropractic Association. Available at: www.jcca-online.org

References

1. Bigos S, Bowyer O, Braen G, et al. Acute Low Back Problems in Adults. *Clinical practice guideline No. 14.* AHCPR Publication No. 95-0642. Rockville, MD: Agency for Health Care Policy and Research, Public Health Service, U.S. Department of Health and Human Services; 1994.

2. Eisenberg D, Kessler R, Foster C, et al. Unconventional medicine in the United States: prevalence, costs and patients. *N Engl J Med.* 1993;328:246–252.

3. Gatterman M, Vernon H. Development of chiropractic nomenclature through consensus. *J Manipulative Physiol Ther.* 1994;7:302–309

4. Lawrence D. Fourteen years of case reports. *J Manipulative Physiol Ther.* 1991; 14:447–449

5. Bergmann T, Peterson D, Lawrence D. *Chiropractic Technique.* New York, NY: Churchill Livingstone; 1989.

6. Shekelle P, Adams A, Chassin M, et al. *The Appropriateness of Spinal Manipulation for Low Back Pain.* Santa Monica, CA: RAND; 1991.

7. Lamm L, Wegner, E., & Collord, D. (1995). Chiropractic scope of practice: what the law allows—update 1993. *J Manipulative Physiol Ther.* 1995;18:16–20.

8. Redwood D. *Contemporary Chiropractic.* New York, NY: Churchill Livingstone; 1997.

9. Haldeman S, ed. *Modern Developments in the Principles and Practice of Chiropractic.* Norwalk, CT: Appleton-Century-Crofts; 1980.

17

Massage Therapy

Audrey E. Snyder, PhD(c), RN, MSN, ACNP-CS

About the Author

Audrey E. Snyder has been a nurse for 21 years. Her past experiences include adult and pediatric intensive care, emergency and flight nursing. She is also a certified massage therapist. She is currently pursuing a doctorate in Nursing at the University of Virginia School of Nursing where her focus is on the integration of complementary and alternative therapies and products. She is working with Dr. Ann Gill Taylor exploring the use of massage on pain and quality of life related symptoms in patients in the acute care environment.

Q: What got you interested in massage therapy?

A: As a critical care, emergency and flight nurse, I saw that many times the treatments used in practice caused pain. I have had a long interest in complementary therapies. My grandmother was a lay midwife and Cherokee Indian. She frequently used herbal and energy therapies for healing. I decided I wanted to learn a hands-on healing therapy to complement my nursing practice. I completed a massage therapy training program and now practice massage in a private practice. Currently I am an associate professor of nursing and nurse practitioner at the University of Virginia and incorporate complementary therapies in my practice and the education provided to our students.

Q: Are there different types of massage therapies?

A: There are different types of massage therapy. Swedish massage underlies most modern massage therapies and has predominantly a relaxation effect. Swedish, deep tissue, and myofasical release techniques were predominate in the training I received. Different massage therapies focus on mechanical, physiologic, reflexive, or mind-body interactions. There are different kinds of specialties such as pregnancy massage, infant massage, and geriatric massage. There are over 80 different methods such as Rolfing, Feldenkrais, Trager, and Alexander Technique. Many massage therapies blend modalities to better address the client's needs. Each of the modalities requires specialized training and many have their own certification requirement. Swedish and deep tissue, or a blend of the two modalities, is the most popular in the United States. Massage often includes other practices that are not exactly massage in a traditional sense, such as polarity therapy, aromatherapy, craniosacral, and manual lymph drainage.

Q: Why do you believe in massage therapy?

A: I believe in massage therapy from my personal and professional experience. Massage is based upon concepts of aiding the body to heal itself. Touch is essential for life. Massage affects the circulatory system, musculoskeltal system, and lymphatic system. I know it has helped me relax and has been beneficial for muscular aches and injuries when massage therapy is received over a period of time. My clients have seen beneficial results in increased mobility of joints, relief of pain and muscle stiffness, and stress reduction.

Q: Does it really work?

A: Yes, it does. Massage promotes health and well being through mechanical changes in body tissues, movement patterns, and physiologic changes at a cellular level in the body. Benefits of massage therapy include
- stress reduction through relaxation and anxiety reduction,
- being more centered and focused with deep breathing,

- promotion of digestion and elimination,
- increased circulation,
- improved lymphatic drainage, and
- increased mobility and range of motion of joints.

Q: What is a massage like?

A: Different types of massage therapy feel different. In general, strokes go toward the heart. Strokes can vary based upon depth, direction, and rhythm. Effleurage or gliding strokes are a major component of Swedish massage. Massage can also incorporate compression, petrissage (kneading), vibration, shaking, rocking, tapotement, friction, joint mobilization, range of motion or stretching. A massage cream, lotion, or oil may facilitate different strokes. A general relaxation session will work on feet, legs, hands, arms, upper shoulders, neck, and back. There are areas of endangerment that are avoided where nerves and blood vessels are close to the skin surface.

Every massage session is unique. An average session lasts 50 minutes to an hour. The massage therapist obtains a medical history, including medications and allergies to medications or topical solutions, and develops an individualized session based upon the client and therapist's mutually agreed goals. The massage therapist relies on the client to provide feedback on strokes, depth, and comfort level. Any area that is being worked upon is appropriately draped with the rest of the body covered. A session may incorporate heat or cold therapy, reflexology, Reiki or other energy therapies, music, and aromatherapy. Massage combines touch with movement. The hands, forearms, elbows, and/or feet of the therapist can be used. Some massage therapist, may use mechanical adjuncts when focusing on a trigger point or an area that is particularly difficult to access. The massage therapist confidentially maintains client history and session information.

Q: How many people use massage therapy?

A: A small percentage of the American public uses massage therapy and this number grows on a yearly basis. In some countries massage is a part of family care. For example in some Asian countries, Thai massage is taught to children at an early age and practiced by all family members. Massage therapy is growing as a result of the increased interest in alternative, natural healing therapies and the growing popularity of spas. For more information, you can go to the American Massage Therapy Association web page available at **http://www.amtamassage.org**.

Q: What is the history of massage?

A: Massage is based in ancient and modern origins. It has been around for thousands of years and has been incorporated into traditional healthcare treatment. Hippocrates was an early proponent of the health benefits of massage. Massage has been steadily used in Eastern medicine, but also has a long Western history. Dr. George Taylor and Dr. Charles Taylor brought it to the United States in the 1850s. It ebbed at the turn of the century and then reemerged in the mid-19th century. Clinics in some areas of Europe and Russia have massage rooms as a part of the medical clinic.

Q: Where does a person get a massage?

A: A person can get a massage in a private massage therapy office, in a physical therapy office, in a spa, in a bed and breakfast, in a chiropractor office, in one's home, in some hospital settings such as cancer treatment centers or labor and delivery units, or seated massage in an airport, or at a health fair. Many healthcare professionals, including nurses, chiropractors, and physicians are trained in massage and incorporate it into their healthcare activities. Massage can be a part of sports training and is incorporated by many professional athletic teams, Olympic squads, and equestrian teams. Over the past few years, massage emergency response teams have emerged as part of a critical incident stress management.

Q: What are some issues related to massage therapy?

A: Some people do not like to be touched. This may have evolved from previous issues with physical or sexual abuse. My husband is also a massage therapist and he has worked with a local sexual assault recovery agency to reintroduce safe touch to these clients. In the early 1900s massage parlors were used as a cover for prostitution. In some places this still exists, for example in Washington, DC, and is widely advertised in popular newspapers such as the Washington Post. This has given massage therapy some negative press. The licensing and certification of massage therapies and research on the benefits of massage therapy has helped to change some of this negative perspective. Most therapists would prefer to not be referred to as a masseuse but as a massage therapist.

Q: What type of research has been done in massage therapy?

A: Dr. Tiffany Fields at the Touch Research Institute in Florida conducted much of the early research in massage therapy. Massage has been shown to be effective in the management of:
- chronic low back pain,[1-4]
- cancer related pain, [5-7]
- migraine headaches,[8-9]
- pain associated with childbirth,[10-14]
- anxiety,[15-18]
- depression,[12,19,20]
- endorphins source,[21-23]
- pre-mature birth,[24-28]
- blood pressure and heart rate,[29,30] and has also been shown to increase the nautral killer cell function.[6,31-33]

Massage has been shown to release endorphins that can modulate pain and mood. Premature infants have shown increased weight gain with massage therapy. Blood pressure and heart rate decrease with massage. Massage can also increase natural killer cell function. The Office of Alternative Medicine at the National Institutes of Health is supporting research in massage and other alternative therapies. More research on the outcomes, benefits, and efficacy of massage is needed.

Q: How much does it cost?

A: Cost varies based on setting and location. In large cities the cost is usually more. In a massage therapy office or spa, cost can range from $45 to $200 for a one hour massage. Prices vary by city and region. In a physical therapy office a 15-minute massage can cost $85.

Q: Does insurance reimburse you for it?

A: In general, insurance does not pay up front or reimburse clients for massage therapy unless it is part of a physical therapy regimen. Insurance companies may have preferred provider contracts that give the client a 10% discount for services. Some car insurance companies will reimburse clients for cost paid up front for massage therapy when it is for specific treatments of injuries with a referral from a physician.

Q: Are there any consequences to my health?

A: It is important for a person receiving a massage to inform the therapist of all medical concerns, medications, herbal therapies, and nutritional supplements. Caution must be used and therapies modified with patients who have a history of diabetes or heart problems. Some consequences of massage may include increased utilization of glucose in diabetics which could possibly contribute to hypoglycemia, and increased venous return to the heart which can result in precipitation of congestive heart failure.

Q: How do I know if it is working and not something else I am doing?

A: Many times massage is not used alone, but as a part of a comprehensive complementary or integrative therapy plan depending on the patient's health condition. Frequently massage may be combined with hydrotherapy, aromatherapy, or be a component of a comprehensive therapy plan with chiropractic, physical therapy, and stretching. They may work synergistically. Massage can be integrated with allopathic medical treatments. Some patients may see a massage therapist prior to a chiropractic adjustment to loosen muscle tension for ease of adjustment or after a chiropractic session to help muscles regain a normal resting state and decrease muscle pain and spasm, which can cause improper alignment of joints.

Q: What will my doctor think about massage therapy?

A: It is important to share your plans to use massage therapy for treatment of a specific problem. Most massage therapists will ask for your written permission to discuss your care with your physician if needed. Many physicians approve of massage therapy for relaxation and for treatment of some specific injuries.

Q: Do I need to approve it with my doctor before I start massage therapy?

A: Massage therapy does not require a doctor's approval. If you have a medical condition you should discuss it with your healthcare provider first.

Q: Will massage therapy hurt me in the long run?

A: Massage therapy should not hurt a person in the long run. With repeated sessions, patients have been shown to have increasing benefits. Patients may become relaxed more quickly with repeated massages and the effects of massage therapy may last longer with repeated exposure. Massage helps with the overall sense of well-being and provides a sense of control for the client.

Q: Are there particular medical conditions that massage is particularly good for treating?

A: Massage is helpful in treating musculoskeletal injuries, chronic and acute pain, hypertension, headaches, temporomandibular joint dysfunction, and stress responses.

Q: Are there any medical conditions where massage should not be used?

A: Massage should not be used when a patient has severe nausea, acute severe pain, or a localized acute injury. Massage should not be performed with open wounds; rashes; or when infection, phlebitis (blood clots), or acute inflammation is present. Massage should not be provided when a client is under the influence of alcohol or recreational drugs. For patients who are on blood thinners, only very light strokes can be performed, if at all. If a client becomes ill with a cold, virus, or bacterial infection just prior to an already scheduled session, a massage therapist will encourage them to reschedule their appointment.

Q: Is there a difference between a therapeutic massage and a massage that one can get at a spa or at a resort?

A: At a spa or resort the focus is generally on relaxation. People may seek out a spa massage to help address sore muscles and other conditions. Many times they turn to spas because it is more business-like, rather than calling a stranger in a phone book. Clients are frequently treating themselves and the massage therapist may only work with this client once. With therapeutic massage the therapist and client set mutual goals for massage therapy and frequently there is more than one session. The therapist and client develop a therapeutic relationship.

Q: Does massage interact with any medications?

A: Massage can increase the effects of antihypertensives and oral hypo-glycemic agents.

Q: Does getting a massage hurt?

A: Some patients may experience temporary pain especially when receiving deep therapy or trigger point work at areas of dysfunction. The massage therapist will obtain feedback from the client to work at a level the client can tolerate.

Q: Are you certified or licensed in what you do?

A: I am certified in the state of Virginia by the Board of Nursing. Currently 30 states and Washington, DC, regulate massage therapists by certification or licensure. The certifying or licensing agency defines the scope of practice for massage therapists. You can check out regulations for your state on the American Massage Therapy Association web page. I am also certified by the National Certification Board for Therapeutic Massage and Bodywork. This certification requires a person to complete the required minimum hours of education and pass a comprehensive exam. It provides proof of qualification to practice. The State Board of Nursing in Virginia requires this certification for state certification as a massage therapist. The states that regulate massage therapy vary widely in which governing body regu-lates massage therapy. There is currently no standard in the field. To main-tain certification as a massage therapist one must complete a minimum number of hours of continuing education, including ethics training, and work a minimum number of hours providing massage therapy.

Q: How long did you go to school to do this?

A: I completed a 500-hour course in therapeutic massage. Some schools now offer full time and part time programs of study ranging from 500–1000 hours of study. Some programs also offer additional training in medical massage. Training for massage therapy usually includes instruction in mas-sage technique as well as in anatomy and physiology, first aid, and ethics.

Q: How can I identify a good massage therapist?

A: Search for a massage therapist who belongs to a professional organization (e.g., American Massage Therapy Association, AMTA), is certified by the National Certification Board for Therapeutic Massage and Bodywork (NCTMB), and is locally certified or licensed. The AMTA has established the Code of Ethics and Standards of Practice for Massage Therapy. The AMTA web site (**www.amtamassage.org**) offers a massage therapist national locator service that lists massage therapists who belong to their organization, or you can call 1-888-THE-AMTA. When a massage therapist joins the AMTA they agree to abide by their code of ethics and standards of practice. The NCTMB certifies massage therapist who pass the national certification exam and maintain their status through continuing education. The NCTMB maintains a list of nationally certified massage therapists available at: **www.nctmb.org**. You can contact the certifying or licensing agency in your state for a list of credentialed providers in your area.

Suggested Readings

National Certification Board for Therapeutic Massage and Bodywork. Available at: http://www.nctmb.org

American Massage Therapy Association. Available at: www.amtamassage.org

American Holistic Nurses Association. Available at: www.ahna.org

American Society for the Alexander Technique. Available at: http://www.alexandertech.com

The Trager Institute available at: http://www.trager.com

Craniosacral Therapy available at: http://upledger.com

Colt GH. See me, feel me, Touch me, heal me. *Life*. 1996;(Sept):35–48.

Colt GH. The magic of touch. *Life*. 1997;(Aug):52–62.

Hayes J, Cox C. Immediate effects of a five-minute foot massage on patients in critical care. *Intensive Crit Care Nurs*. 1999;15(2):77–82.

Smith, MC, Stallings MA, Mariner S, Burrall M. Benefits of massage therapy for hospitalized patients: descriptive and qualitative evaluation. *Altern Ther*. 1999; 5(4):64–71.

Wilkinson S, Aldridge J, Salmon I, Cain E, Wilson B. An evaluation of aromatherapy massage in palliative care. *Palliat Med*. 1999;13(5):409–17.

Zeitlin D, Keller S, Shiflett S, Schleifer S, Bartlett J. Immunological Effects of Massage therapy during academic stress. *Psychosom Med*. 2000;62(1):83.

References

1. Hernandez-Reif M, Field T, Krasnegor J, Theakston H. Lower back pain is reduced and range of motion increased after massage therapy. *Int J Neurosci*. 2001;106(3–4):131–145.

2. Melancon B, Miller LH. Massage therapy versus traditional therapy for low back pain relief: implications for holistic nursing practice. *Holistic Nurs Prac*. 2005; 19(3):116–121.

3. Clare HA, Adams R, Maher CG. A systematic review of efficacy of McKenzie therapy for spinal pain. *Aus J Physio*. 2004;50(4):209–216.

4. Walach H, Guthlin C, Konig M. Efficacy of massage therapy in chronic pain: a pragmatic randomized trial. *J Altern Complement Med*. 2003;9(6):837–846.

5. Pasternack I. Aroma therapy and massage for relieving symptoms of cancer patients. *Duodecim*. 2004;120(22):2694; discussion 2695.

6. Hernandez-Reif M, Field T, Ironson G, et al. Natural killer cells and lymphocytes increase in women with breast cancer following massage therapy. *Intern J Neurosci*. 2005;115(4):495–510.

7. Cassileth BR, Vickers AJ. Massage therapy for symptom control: outcome study at a major cancer center. *J Pain Symptom Manage*. 2004;28(3):244–249.

8. Bag B, Karabulut N. Pain-relieving factors in migraine and tension-type headache. *Int J Clin Pract*. 2005;59(7):760–763.

9. Foster KA, Liskin J, Cen S, et al. The Trager approach in the treatment of chronic headache: a pilot study. *Altern Ther Health Med.* 2004;10(5):40–46.

10. Wang SM, DeZinno P, Fermo L, et al. Complementary and alternative medicine for low-back pain in pregnancy: a cross-sectional survey. *J Altern Complemen Med.* 2005;11(3):459–464.

11. Ingram J, Domagala C, Yates S. The effects of shiatsu on post-term pregnancy. *Complemen Ther Med.* 2005;13(1):11–15.

12. Field T, Diego MA, Hernandez-Reif M, Schanberg S, Kuhn C. Massage therapy effects on depressed pregnant women. *J Psychosom Obstet Gynecol.* 2004;25(2): 115–122.

13. Hinz B. Perineal massage in pregnancy. *J Midwifery Womens Health.* 2005;50(1): 63–64.

14. Spencer KM. The primal touch of birth. Midwives, mothers and massage. *Midwifery Today.* 2004;(70):11–13.

15. McCaffrey R, Taylor N. Effective anxiety treatment prior to diagnostic cardiac catheterization. *Holistic Nurs Pract.* 2005;19(2):70–73.

16. Simmons D, Chabal C, Griffith J, Rausch M, Steele B. A clinical trial of distraction techniques for pain and anxiety control during cataract surgery. *Insight.* 2004;29(4):13–16.

17. Mok E, Woo CP. The effects of slow-stroke back massage on anxiety and shoulder pain in elderly stroke patients. *Complemen Ther Nurs Midwifery.* 2004;10(4):209–216.

18. Goffaux-Dogniez C, Vanfraechem-Raway R, Verbanck P. Appraisal of treatment of the trigger points associated with relaxation to treat chronic headache in the adult: Relationship with anxiety and stress adaptation strategies. *Encephale.* 2003;29(5):377–390. Erratum appears in: *Encephale.* 2004;30(1):94

19. McDougall GJ. Research review: the effect of acupressure with massage on fatigue and depression in patients with end-stage renal disease. *Geriatr Nurs.* 2005;26(3):164–165.

20. Okamoto A, Kuriyama H, Watanabe S, et al. The effect of aromatherapy massage on mild depression: a pilot study. *Psychiatry Clin Neurosci.* 2005;59(3):363.

21. Yang Z, Jiang H. Investigation on analgesic mechanism of acupoint finger-pressure massage on lumbago. *J Tradit Chin Med.* 1994;14(1):35–40.

22. Kaada B, Torsteinbo O. Increase of plasma beta-endorphins in connective tissue massage. *Gen Pharmacol.* 1989;20(4):487–489.

23. Day JA, Mason RR, Chesrown SE. Effect of massage on serum level of beta-endorphin and beta-lipotropin in healthy adults. *Phys Ther.* 1987;67(6):926–930.

24. Diego MA, Field T, Hernandez-Reif M. Vagal activity, gastric motility, and weight gain in massaged preterm neonates. *J Pediatr.* 2005;147(1):50–55.

25. Aly H, Moustafa MF, Hassanein SM, Massaro AN, Amer HA, Patel K. Physical activity combined with massage improves bone mineralization in premature infants: a randomized trial. *J Perinatol.* 2004;24(5):305–309.

26. Vickers A, Ohlsson A, Lacy JB, Horsley A. Massage for promoting growth and development of preterm and/or low birth-weight infants. *Cochrane Database Syst Rev.* 2004(2):CD000390.

27. Dieter JN, Field T, Hernandez-Reif M, Emory EK, Redzepi M. Stable preterm infants gain more weight and sleep less after five days of massage therapy. *J Pediatr Psychol.* 2003;28(6):403–411.

28. Beachy JM. Premature infant massage in the NICU. *Neonatal Net.* 2003;22(3): 39–45.

29. Moyer CA, Rounds J, Hannum JW. A meta-analysis of massage therapy research. *Psychol Bull.* 2004;130(1):3–18.

30. Weerapong P, Hume PA, Kolt GS. The mechanisms of massage and effects on performance, muscle recovery and injury prevention. *Sports Med.* 2005;35(3): 235–256.

31. Hernandez-Reif M, Ironson G, Field T, et al. Breast cancer patients have improved immune and neuroendocrine functions following massage therapy. *J Psychosom Res.* 2004;57(1):45–52.

32. Goodfellow LM. The effects of therapeutic back massage on psychophysiologic variables and immune function in spouses of patients with cancer. *Nurs Res.* 2003;52(5):318–328.

33. Diego MA, Field T, Hernandez-Reif M, Shaw K, Friedman L, Ironson G. HIV adolescents show improved immune function following massage therapy. *Int J Neurosci.* 2001;106(1–2):35–45.

18

Acupuncture and Acupressure

Virginia Hisghman, PhD(c), AP, LAc, MSOM

About the Author

Virginia Hisghman is a predoctoral research fellow at the Center for the Study of Complementary and Alternative Therapies at the University of Virginia in Charlottesville, Virginia. Her background in Oriental medicine includes training in both Traditional Chinese Medicine and Traditional Japanese Medicine. She has served as the assistant dean of academics at the Texas College of Traditional Chinese Medicine. She has served as a site visitor and commissioner (practitioner member) for the Accreditation Commission for Acupuncture and Oriental Medicine. She is a member of the Society of Acupuncture Research and the American Organization of Bodywork Therapies of Asia research committee.

...;ot you interested in acupuncture and acupressure?

A: ...me interested in Oriental medicine in the early 1980s after being treated for stress by an acupuncturist. Much to my amazement the acupuncture worked, and there were no side effects. The effectiveness of the treatment was so intriguing that I began an exploration of alternative medicine that has continued for over two decades.

Q: Why is acupuncture and acupressure considered Complementary and Alternative Medicine (CAM)?

A: Both of these modalities deal with all aspects of the patient's life including lifestyle, diet, relationships, emotional issues, physical health, and overall well being which is a holistic approach to health people are seeking.[1] An estimated 30% to 50% of the adult population in the United States is using alternative therapies and products.[2] The trend now is to integrate allopathic and CAM for the benefit of the patient in order to provide a wider range of safe and effective options in health care.

Q: How many people use acupuncture and acupressure?

A: Complementary and alternative therapy usage has increased in the United States almost 45% from 1990 to 1997, with an estimated 629 million visits to CAM providers. This exceeded the total number of visits to primary care physicians. An estimated $21 billion was spent annually for CAM professional services.[3] These are staggering statistics and we must acknowledge that the public demand for alternative medicine is rapidly increasing.

Q: What is the difference between acupressure and acupuncture?

A: Both systems theorize that the vital life force, or Qi, follows preset pathways (meridians) and can be accessed to improve circulation of Qi by acupuncture points (acupoints) located along the meridians. In healthy individuals Qi flows freely and unobstructed, however, obstructions or stagnation of Qi can result in health problems. Acupuncture and acupressure restore the flow and balance of Qi in the body. Acupuncture utilizes sterile, disposable needles that are inserted into acupoints at specific depths. With acupressure, the practitioner does a pressing action with a finger, hand, elbow, or specialized instrument to stimulate the acupoint to promote circulation of the Qi.

Q: Why do you believe in acupuncture and acupressure?

A: From personal experience and as a licensed acupuncturist, I have objective experience that Oriental medicine is effective, whether the patient believes in it or not. Each year millions of people receive acupuncture or acupressure treatment and benefit from them. In 1998–1999, Congress mandated that research would be done to address the mechanism of action of this alternative therapy.[4] Since then, a tremendous increase in funded research done at major universities has shown its efficacy in randomized clinical trials.

Q: How is acupressure different from massage therapy?

A: Acupressure is very targeted and specific in its application because it uses the meridians and acupoints to treat the condition. Depending on the patient's chief complaint, a specific acupressure protocol is formulated to stimulate the appropriate acupoints and meridians. The ultimate goal is to restore balance in the body. Massage therapies focus on different treatment principles.

Q: How does it work?

A: Qi (Chinese) or ki (Japanese), pronounced chi (chee), is the word that describes the vital life force. The life force animates the human body and encompasses the physical, spiritual, emotional, and mental components of the individual. Qi flows through the meridians and to the degree that the Qi is strong, free flowing, and balanced the individual is healthy. If the Qi is weak, obstructed, excessive, or out of balance, the person will have less than optimal health. The purpose of either acupuncture or acupressure is to regulate, harmonize, balance, and strengthen the Qi in the body using needles or acupressure of acupoints along the meridians.

Q: Are there different styles of acupuncture?

A: Yes, there are four major acupuncture styles practiced in the United States: Traditional Chinese Medicine (TCM), Traditional Japanese Medicine (TJM), Tibetan Medicine, and Korean Medicine. There are also numerous related acupuncture therapies such as Auricular Acupuncture, which is very effective in treating addictions. Electro-acupuncture is another treatment used to reduce pain relief that uses a small amount of electrical stimulation on the needles from a unit similar to a Transcutaneous Electrical Nerve Stimulation (TENS) device.

Q: How do I know which type is right for me?

A: The styles and treatment protocols vary greatly between the four systems and you should discuss this issue with your alternative healthcare provider. There is an abundance of information available in books and on the Internet on these various modalities. I always recommend that the patient be well informed of the modality the practitioner will be using.

Q: What will treatments be like?

A: The practitioner will do an assessment of your chief complaint, determine a diagnosis, and formulate a treatment plan. Single use, sterile needles will be used in accordance with good clinical hygienic practices and inserted into acupuncture points. The needles vary in size, width of the shaft, metal composition, and the shape of the head. Most often they are stainless steel and are less than the size of a human hair in width. Usually there is little or no painful sensation felt by the patient when the needle is inserted. When patients do feel the needle being inserted, they sometimes describe the sensation as similar to the feeling of a mosquito bite. There are several sensations that the patient will feel when the Qi arrives to the acupoint which is called deQi (pronounced dah-chee). It can be the feeling of numbness, a tingling sensation, a dull and achy feeling, or heaviness in the area. All these sensations will dissipate as the treatment continues. In acupressure, the practitioner will do a similar assessment and formulate a treatment plan for the patient. The patient will feel a pressing sensation and sometimes an achy feeling when an acupoint is being stimulated by the practitioner.

Acupuncture and acupressure are holistic practices and your practitioner will be working with you on improving many areas in your life that may be contributing to your condition. Therefore, practical suggestions may be discussed to help improve these areas. It is the goal of Oriental medicine to treat the root cause of the condition and strengthen internal resistance to disease by restoring optimal balance of Qi. Most patients report a difference after their first treatment. Your health, quality of life, and outlook should all improve as you continue your treatment program.

Q: Is there any risk to me?

A: Risks associated with acupuncture include fainting from needle insertion, bruising, bleeding, infection at site of insertion, hematoma, pain when needle is inserted, and transmission of disease due to unhygienic practices. Risk of transmission of disease to the patient with the use of disposable needles is rare. There is a minimal chance of these side effects from acupuncture as demonstrated in safety studies.[5-9] Depending on the state, the patient will sign a document stating that the risks have been explained prior to commencing treatment.

Q: How often will I need treatments?

A: Most patients start with one or two treatments per week and then taper off as their condition improves. Chronic conditions usually will require more treatments than acute conditions. Eight to ten treatments is considered a course of treatments and depending on the severity of the illness, a patient will require several courses of treatment.

Q: What type of research has been done?

A: The continued increase of consumer demand in the United States for CAM led Congress to establish the National Center for Complementary and Alternative Medicine (NCCAM) in 1998 at the National Institutes of Health (NIH). NCCAM has been tasked with the responsibility of ensuring rigorous and evidence-based research on CAM. CAM research centers are now found in major universities. Acupuncture is among the most researched of all CAM. These studies have been conducted in conditions such as osteoarthritis, back pain, painful menses, migraine headaches, depression, fibromyalgia, post chemotherapy nausea and insomia. Acupuncture is currently being studied with individualized treatment protocols in blinded, randomized, placebo/sham, and controlled trials.

Q: How much does acupuncture and acupressure cost?

A: Treatment costs for acupuncture range from $60 to $125 per session. Acupressure sessions will cost approximately $60 to $80 per session.

Q: Does insurance reimburse you for it?

A: A survey done by the Kaiser Family Foundation and Health Research and Educational Trust found insurance coverage for acupuncture is increasing. The employer coverage for acupuncture increased 14% from 2002 to 2004.[10] Insurance coverage varies from state to state, so check with the individual insurance company on coverage.

Q: What will my doctor think about this?

A: More doctors are recommending that their patients use acupuncture or acupressure and are actively working with acupuncturists to treat patients in a holistic approach to care.

Q: Do I need to approve it with my doctor before I start using it?

A: Each state varies on this issue and your practitioner should be aware of the state requirements. In states such as Florida, acupuncturists are classified as primary care providers and you will not need your doctor's approval before receiving treatments. In other states, you may need to have been examined for the condition being treated by a physician, a doctor of osteopathy, or a doctor of chiropractic medicine in the previous 12 months with some exceptions such as smoking, pain relief, and weight loss.

Q: Does it interact with any of my medications I am taking?

A: Acupuncture alone doesn't interact with medications, but some of the herbal formulas prescribed by the practitioner could. There are particular acupoints and associated treatments that are contraindicated for certain medical conditions. For example, electro-acupuncture would not be used with a patient who has a pacemaker and certain acupoints are contraindicated for pregnant women.

Q: What type of training and requirements are needed to become a licensed acupuncturist? certified in acupressure?

A: A degree from an accredited Oriental medical college in the United States and a four-year master's level program. A minimum of 60 undergraduate hours from an accredited university or college are required before admission into the program. American Organization for Bodywork Therapies of Asia training for Oriental bodywork takes approximately two years to complete.

Acupuncturists in most states are required to pass a national board examination to be certified to practice as Diplomates in Acupuncture and Chinese Herbology. This is regulated by the National Certification Commission for Acupuncture and Oriental Medicine (NCCAOM) that is tasked with the "mission of promoting nationally recognized standards of competence and safety in acupuncture and Oriental Medicine and for the purpose of protecting the public from unsafe practices. It is a considerable professional achievement to earn the designation 'Diplomate in Acupuncture' (NCCAOM). NCCAOM Certification indicates to employers, patients, and peers that one has met national standards for the safe and competent practice of acupuncture as defined by the profession."[11] In addition to the national boards, each state has specific regulations for licensure to practice. Individual state Acupuncture Board practice acts, requirements, and regulations can easily be obtained through the Internet in the state government sites. For acupressure, a similar NCCAOM board examination is now required of practitioners to be certified as Diplomates in Asian Bodywork Therapy.

Q: How do I find a qualified practitioner in my area? How can I find out if my practitioner is qualified or licensed to do acupuncture?

A: Most states have an Acupuncture Board whose duty is to protect the public and ensure the qualifications of its members. Each regulating board has lists of licensed acupuncturists and, similar to other healthcare professions, information is available in regards to complaints or malpractice. At the NCCAOM website (**http://nccaom.org**) you can search for practitioners who have a Diplomate designation under the "Find a Practitioner" icon.*

---

*This chapter was supported in part by Grant Number T32AT00052 from the National Center for Complementary and Alternative Medicine (NCCAM), National Institutes of Health, and its contents are solely the responsibility of the authors and do not necessarily represent the official views of the NCCAM or the National Institutes of Health.

Suggested Readings

Beinfeld H, Korngold E. *Between Heaven and Earth: A Guide to Chinese Medicine.* 1st ed. New York, NY: Ballantine Books; 1991.

Kaptchuk TJ. *The Web That Has No Weaver: Understanding Chinese Medicine.* New York, NY: Congdon & Weed; 1983.

Pearson P. *An Introduction to Acupuncture: A Practical Guide for GPs and Other Medical Personnel.* Surry, England: Medical Centre; 1987.

Stux G, Pomeranz B. *Acupuncture: Textbook and Atlas: With 98 Figures and an Acupuncture Selector.* Sahm KA, translator; Kopen P, illustrator. New York, NY: Springer-Verlag; 1987.

Worsley JR. *Traditional Chinese Acupuncture.* Shaftesbury, England: Element Books; 1982

National Certification Commission for Acupuncture and Oriental Medicine. Available at: http://nccaom.org

American Organization for Bodywork Therapies of Asia. Available at: www.aobta.org

Council of Colleges of Acupuncture and Oriental Medicine. Available at: www.ccaom.org

American Association of Oriental Medicine. Available at: www.aaom.org

United States Library of Medicine. Available at: www.nlm.nih.gov/archive/20040823/pubs/cbm/acupuncture.html

References

1. Astin J. Why patients use alternative medicine: results of a national survey. *JAMA. 1999;279:*1548–1583.

2. Landmark Healthcare *The Landmark Report: Public Perception of Alternative Care.* Sacramento, CA: Landmark Healthcare; 1998.

3. Eisenberg D, Davis R, Etner S, Appel S, Wilkey S, Van Rompay M, Kessler R. Trends in alternative medicine use in the United States, 1990–1997. *JAMA.* 1998;280(18):1569–1575.

4. National Institutes of Health (NIH). NIH consensus development conference on acupuncture program and abstract. Bethesda, MD: National Institutes of Health; 1997.

5. Lao L, Hamilton G, Fu J, Berman B. Is acupuncture safe? A systematic review of case reports. *Altern Ther Health Med.* 2003;9(1):72–83.

6. MacPherson H, Thomas K, Walters S, Fitter M. The York acupuncture safety study: prospective survey of 34,000 treatments by traditional acupuncturists. *BMJ.* 2001;323(7311):486–487.

7. Ernst F, White A. Prospective studies of the safety of acupuncture: a systematic review. *Am J Med.* 2001;110(6):481–485.

8. Yamashita H, Tsukayama H, Tanno Y, Nishijo K. Adverse events in acupuncture and moxibustion treatment: a six-year survey at a national clinic in Japan. *J Altern Complement Med.* 1999;5(3):229–236.

9. Melchart D, Weidenhammer W, Streng A, Reitmayr S, Hoppe A, Ernst E, Linde K. Prospective investigation of adverse effects of acupuncture in 97,733 patients. *Arch Intern Med.* 2004;164(1);104–105.

10. Henry J. Kaiser Family Foundation. Employer Health Benefits 2004 Annual Survey. Chicago, IL: Health Research and Educational Trust.

11. National Certification Commission for Acupuncture and Oriental Medicine. Available at: htttp://www.nccaom.org/aboutus.htm. Accessed on August 15, 2005.

19

Taiji (T'ai Chi)

John Alton, BA, MFA

About the Author

John Alton is the author of *Living Qigong* and *Unified Fitness*. He has over 30 years experience in East Asian martial arts and is currently the only non-Chinese Westerner mainland China officially recognizes as an authentic Qigong master. He currently heads Unified Fitness, LLC, a research and development company that focuses on the roles of the immune system and infection in multi-factorial or unknown cause disease.

Q: What is Taiji (T'ai Chi)?

A: The terms *Taiji* or *T'ai Chi* come from the longer expressions *Taijiquan* or *T'ai Chi Ch'uan*. The longer expressions are usually translated as supreme, ultimate fist and refer to a martial arts exercise routine. The abbreviated expressions *Taiji* or *T'ai Chi* also refer to the Daoist (also written as Taoist) yin/yang symbol: a circle divided into light and dark halves, separated by a curved line. The term *Taiji* or *T'ai Chi* refers to that curved line, which marks the supreme boundary that separates all opposites, such as light and darkness, hard and soft, hot and cold, life and death. Thus, Taiji or T'ai Chi is an exercise that puts the practitioner in touch with this great boundary.

In practice, Taiji is a form of Chinese martial art that consists of slow-motion strikes, blocks, kicks, and evasions. History credits the formalization of this martial art to a 17th-century man named Chen. In subsequent centuries, others built upon, expanded, and contracted the so-called Chen style into a myriad of styles, each bearing the name of its innovator. This fragmentation and multiplication of styles continued until the People's Republic of China began standardizing Taiji in the late 1950s and early 1960s for both competition and clarification. Today on the mainland there are four predominant systems of Taiji: Chen, Yang, Wu, and Sun, each named after its founder. Of the four, the Yang style is the most widely recognized and practiced.

Q: Are the movements of Taiji organized in a certain way?

A: Each Taiji maneuver is numbered and arranged in a choreographed sequence that can take only a few minutes to over half an hour to complete. Typically, the number of movements in the choreographed sequences, which are generally referred to as forms, serve in part to name the Taiji routine. Twenty-four-step, Thirty-six-step, Forty-two-step, Forty-eight-step, Eighty-eight-step, and One-hundred-twenty-six-step are some examples of numbered names of Taiji forms that enjoy widespread popularity.

Q: How does Taiji differ from other forms of exercise?

A: In addition to slow movement, relaxation of the upper body and meticulous focus on lower body mechanics distinguish Taiji from other forms of exercise. During a Taiji form, the practitioner keeps the muscles of the chest, back, shoulders, neck, and arms soft and relaxed, while the waist, hips, and legs do most of the work. Waist, hip, and leg movements cause the body's weight to shift continuously. For several seconds at a time, one leg will bear all the body's weight, while gluteal and hip muscles lift and reposition the non-weight-bearing leg. In this way, Taiji is able to focus on and tone the so-called core: muscles deep in the trunk, abdomen, and pelvis that are necessary for sustained power, stability, and resilience.

Q: **How is breathing used in Taiji?**

A: Another aspect of Taiji that sometimes gets ignored in favor of musculoskeletal mechanics is breathing. In traditional Taiji, breathing is extremely important for maintaining health. Sometimes breathing technique is taught in a separate class under the label of *Qigong* (Ch'i Kung), which means breath work.

Q: **What is the difference between the term** *Qi* **in Qigong and the term** *Chi* **in T'ai Chi?**

A: The confusion here is the result created by two competing systems for transliterating Chinese ideograms (word pictures) into Romanized letters that Western people can understand. One system is called Wade-Giles, which is where the T'ai Chi spelling comes from. The other is called Pinyin (pronounced pen-yen), which is where the Taiji spelling comes from. Though Wade-Giles is an earlier system, Westerners devised it. The Peoples Republic of China created the Pinyin system to clear up misunderstandings created by Wade-Giles.

The term *Tai* or in Wade-Giles *T'ai,* means great or extreme. Literally the term translates as too, as in *too* hard. While the difference between the two systems appears small in this case, the situation changes with the second portion of the word. The term *ji* not only looks much different from *chi,* but also means something entirely different if Wade-Giles pronunciation rules are poorly understood, which is often the case. *Ji* means boundary or extreme, which is what the Wade-Giles expression *chi* also means. Both terms should be pronounced jee, as in jeep. But once the Wade-Giles spelling became commonplace in locations like San Francisco and New York, Wade-Giles pronunciation rules—which rely heavily on the use of apostrophes to vary pronunciation—fell into obscurity. Eventually, the term *chi* got confused with the Wade-Giles expression for life force, *ch'i,* which is pronounced chee. In Pinyin, the same word is spelled *qi.*

To avoid such confusion and to honor China's historical ownership of the practice, I use the Pinyin spelling and encourage those mired in the confusion created by misuse of the Wade-Giles system to follow mainland China's lead.

Q: **What is the main difference between Taiji practiced in mainland China and in the rest of the world?**

A: The key difference between the Taiji practiced in mainland China and everywhere else, is that China has standardized Taiji to the extent that the West has standardized football, basketball, and baseball. In fact, the Ministry of Sport, a government cabinet post, oversees the standardization process. The Ministry of Sport created a college curriculum for martial arts, taught in state-sponsored martial arts colleges throughout China. These martial arts colleges award undergraduate, masters, and doctoral degrees in Taiji and martial arts.

In the United States. and most everywhere else, Taiji instruction has no standardization. Instead, self-defined Taiji masters offer instruction in small schools or community recreation programs. These instructors can vary wildly in terms of their knowledge and ability. The novice has little way of knowing the quality of Taiji instruction. In former years, proof of family traditions lineages and impressive martial skill were the only way to show the public the level of quality offered by a particular instructor. Now, affiliation with or recognition by official Chinese sources is a good indication of competence and level of sophistication.

Q: What are the benefits of combining Qigong with Taiji exercise?

A: Qigong is largely a meditative breathing and sensory skill, but it can also incorporate Taiji-like subtle movement. The routine offered in my own school combines all three: breathing, sensory meditation, and subtle movement. I have studied a number of systems over the years and have found that the combination works most quickly and effectively.

Qigong can boost the immune system and produce a deep state of relaxation. The inclusion of Qigong in a Taiji program is a good sign, but, like Taiji, Qigong looks deceptively simple. In fact, without a clear program it is extremely difficult to master. Therefore, prospective Taiji or Qigong students should look closely at the instructor and listen to the claims of long-standing students.

Q: How important are the instructor's apparent health and physical prowess?

A: Taiji and Qigong are health-promoting exercises, and if physical or psychological problems show in the instructor(s), then skill level is probably lacking. If an instructor is infirm, and he or she is teaching under the auspices of a more advanced, healthier teacher, then instructor fitness is less of a concern.

If an instructor is relatively young, he or she should be able to perform Taiji at a substantial athletic level. Their stances should be low and their kicks high. With older instructors, especially former martial arts athletes whose bodies are put under stresses and strains along the lines of Olympic gymnasts, a lack of athleticism in their Taiji movements should be less of a concern.

Q: What should a beginner know about the instructor before beginning training?

A: Find out about the instructor's training history. Though Taiji instructors often boast an impressive lineage in terms of their Taiji training, the information is often lost on the novice, who knows little (and perhaps cares even less) about such details. The amount of time spent under the direct scrutiny of a high-level teacher, versus once a week instruction or instruction under a student of the high-level teacher, are important considerations in assessing how much weight to give to an instructor's training credentials. Publications and awards are good signs, but don't necessarily guarantee quality instruction. Sometimes award-winning or book-wielding teachers develop a distaste for actual teaching, which they relegate to students.

Generally speaking, a Taiji instructor should have studied at least two years on a more or less daily basis with a high-level Taiji instructor to qualify as someone who can single-handedly lead a class.

Q: Since Taiji is practiced slowly and softly, is it easy to learn?

A: Because Taiji looks easy, due to the soft, fluid-looking movements, many are completely blindsided when they find out the exercise is hard, sometimes frustrating work. In some ways, Taiji is more demanding than conventional Western exercise because it forces you to think carefully about discrete movements most people never pay attention to. Moreover, the strain of having to think so meticulously about weight distribution, foot position, and hip, knee, and ankle angles sometimes taxes the mind to the point of being stressful. In taking up Taiji, the novice must be prepared for a long, slow, learning process.

Q: Are all Taiji programs the same, or do they differ from one another?

A: There are at least three key ways that Taiji programs can differ. The first and most obvious way has to do with the style of Taiji being taught. Remember that there are at least four official styles recognized in mainland China, and historically there are many more. Though similar in many ways, some, such as the Chen and Yang styles, can differ considerably in terms of not only technique, but also speed and power.

The second key way Taiji programs can differ is in their emphasis on the martial aspect of the exercise. Many of the most popular forms have retained their original fighting focus, and this means some of the movements might be physically challenging. A program for senior citizens should be pared down and divested of such movements; conversely, a program that proposes to teach authentic Taiji should include the more difficult movements, as well as martial interpretations of the movements.

A third factor affecting Taiji programs is the instructor. Every individual colors Taiji in some fashion. A strong, athletic instructor is likely to make Taiji as challenging as possible, whereas an elderly or less athletic instructor is apt to emphasize subtlety and relaxation over athleticism.

Q: Why has the Western medical community begun to advocate Taiji for seniors in recent years?

A: In 1995, the *Journal of the American Medical Association* published a study that showed that Taiji practice was better than any other exercise at decreasing the risk of falling in the elderly.[1] This finding supported previous data that showed the major immediate benefits of practicing Taiji include greater lower body strength, improved peripheral circulation, and increased bone density. More studies have confirmed these results.[2,3] These combined considerations make Taiji the optimum exercise for a senior population. In mainland China, millions of seniors use Taiji to help them stay healthy and in shape. Thus Western medicine is finally coming around to embracing what the far East has known for many years.

Q: Are there any particular areas of the body that Taiji puts under special strain?

A: In practicing Taiji, the trouble areas to watch out for are the lower back, the hips (pelvis), and knees. Taiji puts a great deal of stress on these parts of the body, and programs should call attention to these potential difficulties and offer those who are impaired in these areas modified versions of the movements so as to prevent injury or further irritation. With careful attention to hip, knee, and foot alignment, however, these problems can be avoided. Practitioners should also be careful not to exceed their skill level, such as stooping too low or kicking too high.

Q: How often do you have to practice to succeed in Taiji?

A: Success in Taiji depends on regular daily practice. Unfortunately, most Taiji classes are conducted on a part-time basis, meeting usually no more than once a week. At such a pace, progress will be very slow, often leading the novice to become frustrated. To reap the full benefit of the practice, students must anticipate putting in at least ten minutes of practice every day.

Q: Are Taiji lessons expensive?

A: If you want quality in your Taiji instruction, expect to pay for it. Institutions and health centers tend to regard Taiji simply as an exercise. In fact, high-level Taiji expertise should be viewed as a form of specialized health knowledge that relatively few people currently understand. Because there are currently no standards for determining quality Taiji instruction (except in mainland China), institutions and health centers are forced to guess at the quality of instructors and offer courses at rock-bottom prices, thus encouraging a tendency to undervalue the practice and to foster continued confusion about instructor quality.

Q: How important are the facilities where the Taiji class is being offered?

A: The quality of training facilities may vary and may have nothing to do with the quality of instruction. Taiji classes held in wellness or fitness centers must compete with aerobics classes and other traditional exercise classes and are thus subject to financial constraints that may affect the quality of the instruction. If the instructor operates a school outside the host center, then you can be a little more assured that the center hasn't hired someone cheaply in order to satisfy what they probably consider a small, in-house demand. Though you may receive slipshod instruction in a less fancy place as readily as in an upscale wellness center, an instructor who has managed to create a full-time, though shabbily kept, Taiji school probably has more to offer than someone who teaches part-time at a gleaming, immaculate facility.

Q: What sort of clothing should be worn when practicing Taiji?

A: Any loose, comfortable clothing, with plenty of waist and legroom, makes good Taiji practice apparel. Traditionally, Taiji practitioners wear silk, which is reputed to enhance the flow of Qi. Also, silk makes the movements look smooth and silky, like the material itself. Purchasing a silk Taiji uniform might accentuate your Taiji practice in several ways. The feel of the material is pleasant. It's also very adaptable to temperature—it breathes in hot weather and retains heat in the cold. It also creates an aura of ritual that can help make practices feel special.

Q: What kind of shoes should be worn when practicing Taiji?

A: Comfortable tennis shoes with flat soles make excellent Taiji footwear. Traditional cloth-soled Taiji shoes offer the same benefits as the traditional silk uniform. But the cloth soles degrade quickly and don't work well outdoors, especially if the ground is moist. Plastic-soled Taiji shoes help solve some of the problem, but they too lack the durability of a good, flat-soled tennis shoe. Most of the Chinese Taiji practitioners I know prefer flat-soled tennis shoes to the traditional Taiji shoe.

Q: Can you learn self-defense from Taiji?

A: Over time a person can learn self-defense from practicing Taiji. This is largely accomplished in two ways. First, the instructor should break down individual movements and demonstrate how they can be used in a self-defense situation. The second way is to practice two-person choreographed routines typically referred to as push-hands. In a simple push-hand routine, two people face each other and press the backs of the same-side hands against one another. One of the people initiates a slow, gentle push, which the other person absorbs by turning the waist and sinking back on the rear leg. Once the pusher has extended the push to the point where his or her center of balance is destabilized, the absorber of the push shifts the weight forward again, turning the waist, and pushing forward, effectively reversing roles in the routine. Likewise, the one who initiated the push responds by absorbing the forward movement of the pusher, until the extension of the push erodes the stability of the pusher, whereupon the roles are reversed again. This reciprocal give and take can go on for as long as the participants want. There are many push-hands routines, some involving dozens of complex, two-person movements that require complicated footwork from the participants. The idea is that the push-hand routines will acclimate the participants to the physics of a violent encounter, to which an automatic push-hands response occurs naturally. In my own experience, the first method of teaching self-defense with Taiji is the more effective of the two approaches, because it is the simplest.

Q: Can Taiji be learned from books and video tapes?

A: I recommend against trying to learn exclusively from books and videos. There is no substitute for a good instructor. Even so, you should ask your instructor if he or she can recommend a complementary book or video to help you learn more thoroughly. Books are the hardest to learn moves from, but they sometimes provide first-rate background information. Videos make excellent tools for learning movement, but they rate a distant second when compared to an excellent flesh-and-blood teacher.

Q: How long does it take to learn a simple Taiji form?

A: If you attend classes three days a week, it should take you no more than a couple of months to learn the Twenty-four-step Yang-style Taiji form. This includes basic training for the foot and hand work, along with breathing patterns. If you are an adept student, you are likely to finish closer toward the second month. The less adept should count on working up till the third month. If you're attending a once-a-week class, and you don't have a learning tool such as a book or video to help you with additional practices, it may take you four months to complete the Twenty-four-step form. Officially, the Twenty-four-step form is the shortest Taiji form, but instructors often invent smaller forms that serve as bridges to longer routines. These smaller forms may take much less time to complete.

Q: What are some immediate heath benefits that come with Taiji practice?

A: Within the first week or so of practice, greater lower body strength and better balance can occur. After about three weeks of steady Taiji workouts, you should begin to feel a greater sense of calm that lingers after exercise sessions. You may feel heaviness or pulsing in the hands that accompanies this sense of calm. If you check your blood pressure, you may find that it has dropped substantially after Taiji (sometimes as much as 20 points). Through continued Taiji practice and Qigong training, these relaxation benefits may flower into full-blown immune system changes that allow you to resist infection and stress. The more you practice, the greater your resistance to infection and stress. This is the grand internal strength the Chinese classics refer to when they write of the health benefits of Taiji. For this reason, the classics consider Taiji a high, spiritual practice that should be practiced daily over the course of one's life.

Suggested Readings

Alton J. *Living Qigong: The Chinese Way to Good Health and Long Life*. Boston, MA: Shambhala Publications; 1997.

Alton J. *Unified Fitness: A 35-Day Exercise Program for Sustainable Health*. Charlottesville, VA: Hampton Roads Publishing; 2002.

References

1. Province MA, Hadley EC, Hornbrook MC, et al. The effects of exercise on falls in elderly patients. A preplanned meta-analysis of the FICSIT Trials. Frailty and Injuries: Cooperative Studies of Intervention Techniques. *JAMA*. 1995;273(17): 1341–1347.

2. Li F, Harmer P, Fisher KJ, McAuley E. Tai Chi: improving functional balance and predicting subsequent falls in older persons. *Med Sci Sports Exer*. 2004;36(12): 2046–2052.

3. Wolf SL, Sattin RW, Kutner M, O'Grady M, Greenspan AI, Gregor RJ. Intense tai chi exercise training and fall occurrences in older, transitionally frail adults: a randomized, controlled trial. *J Amer Geriatr Soc*. 2003;51(12):1693–1701.

20

Reiki

Kathleen A. Lipinski, RN, MSN

About the Author

Kathleen A. Lipinski is a Holistic nurse in private practice on Long Island, New York. She is a full time Reiki Master Teacher, and has taught Reiki at nursing schools and community colleges as well as traveling to various states. She is a senior licensed teacher with the International Center for Reiki Training as well as the president and founder of the Long Island Reiki Connection, a nonprofit resource and support group for Reiki Practitioners. More information is available at **www.longislandreikiconnection.org**.

Q: What got you interested in Reiki? How long have you been practicing Reiki?

A: I attended a workshop for nurses on energy healing in 1992. Everyone was talking about this new technique called Reiki. After my first experience with energy healing, I was hooked. So I inquired about Reiki and found a teacher through a friend. The rest is history.

I took my first Reiki class later that same year and have been using it every day since. I completed my Reiki Master Teacher training in 1994 and started teaching right away.

Q: Describe to me what a Reiki session would be like.

A: A Reiki session is ideally conducted in a quiet room, where the person is sitting in a chair or lying on a Reiki or massage table. The quiet setting is conducive to relaxation but is not always necessary. Reiki is done anywhere and anytime, in a hospital bed, on an operating room table, in a person's bed at home, in a wheelchair, or wherever the person is. Soft, gentle, relaxing music is played in the background. A general session, or full body, includes placing hands on or just above 12–16 positions on the body. These positions are generally located near the major organs of the body. This includes the head, the front and the back of the body. The person receiving Reiki is asked to quiet their mind, focus inward, and allow themselves to receive this relaxing, healing energy.

A Reiki session can be focused on just one or two areas of concern, injury, pain, or discomfort. The session is as long or as short as needed lasting 10–40 minutes, to a full body session lasting 45–90 minutes. Talking is usually not encouraged so the person can receive the full benefits of relaxation. Deep relaxation and feelings of peace and calm are reported most often from those that receive Reiki.

Q: Why do you believe in Reiki? Have your beliefs changed over the years?

A: I believe in Reiki because of the results I have seen, the experiences I have had giving and receiving Reiki, and the experiences that people have reported to me. My basic beliefs have remained the same but my overall beliefs about Reiki have expanded. When I first studied Reiki, I thought it was simply a hands-on healing technique. After 13 years of practicing and teaching Reiki, I now know that it can be much more than a simple technique. Over time, Reiki becomes a way of life: the way of the compassionate heart.

Q: What is Reiki and where does the name Reiki originate?

A: I would start by saying that Reiki is an energy in itself; it is the energy of the life force that animates all living things. One can feel it and some can see it. Some are beginning to find ways to measure it and observe its effects. "Rei" means universal and "Ki" is life force energy. Therefore, Reiki is universal life force energy. Martial arts, Tai Chi, and Qigong are all practices that are based on the flow of chi or the life force energy. Eastern practices are aware of the flow of chi and how to balance and maintain it to promote health. There are various forms of Reiki named after the founder or the way of doing Reiki. Such examples are Usui Reiki, Tibetan Reiki, and White Light Reiki.

Q: What are the Reiki Ideals and how is spirituality connected to these concepts?

A: Reiki can be a spiritual path for some. I have to add here that Reiki is not about religion. One can continue to believe in and practice their religion of choice and still do Reiki. Spiritual refers to the spirit of the person, who they are at the center of their being. Keep in mind that the choice of how to use Reiki and incorporate it into one's life is an individual one. Some people choose only to explore the hands-on healing aspects of Reiki.

The Reiki Ideals are the foundation of this spiritual path. Dr. Usui, the founder of Reiki, gave them to his patients and students. They are guidelines on how to live one's life and balance body, mind, and spirit. They are based on the premise of "Just for Today . . ." promoting the art of being totally aware of, focused, and present in this moment. Thus the Reiki Ideals are a guide for letting go of worry and anger. They remind one to be grateful for all people and things in their life. They promote continual work on healing oneself. The Reiki Ideals promote compassion and kindness towards all living things.

Q: How is Reiki used as energy to empower the person?

A: Reiki can be a self-empowerment tool. When someone works with energy, their awareness is expanded and they learn that the world we live in is an energy-based world. Looking at the world and how it functions as energy gives us an entirely new perspective on life and how to live it. A person can see that things are more than they seem. Situations have an energy; relationships, animals, plants, and food have energy. One also begins to understand that emotions are energy.

This empowers a person and helps them to understand that they can affect their world and events in a positive or negative fashion. The more you do Reiki, the more you understand energy. You learn to read it, tap into it, sense it, feel it, and then apply or work with it. Thus Reiki can be used for healing and balancing all aspects of life. It is important to note that Reiki cannot do harm; it can only be used for good. It cannot be used to control people or things.

Reiki also nourishes the spirit of the person and helps them to keep on keeping on. It also enhances natural abilities. It helps one to develop and enhance all their senses. Thus it is a very powerful self-care and self-empowerment tool, helping a person to become all they can and are meant to be. Just think of continuously receiving life force energy—a constant deposit in one's energy bank!

Q: Does Reiki really work? What can it be used for?

A: Yes. Reiki addresses the totality of a person, body, mind, and spirit and can be used for many things:

- Relaxation;
- Balancing body, mind, and spirit;
- Restoration of vitality; enhancement of well-being;
- Relief from physical and emotional effects of stress;
- Recovery from injuries, surgery, trauma, chemotherapy, and radiation;
- Relief from pain, anxiety, and emotional states;
- Preparing (strengthening and balancing) the body for surgery, medical procedures, chemotherapy, radiation, etc.;
- Acceleration of the body's healing process;
- Promotion of a healthy pregnancy and childbirth;
- Enhancement of immune system or immune response;
- Eases and comforts during the dying process;
- Calming and nurturing; and
- Self-care (helps prevent burnout).

Reiki can be used for persons of all ages; from before birth (*in utero*) throughout the life span. Animals also love Reiki and many pet owners, horse trainers, and veterinarians now offer or get Reiki for their pets.

Q: Can anyone explain how it works?

A: As a Reiki Master Teacher, I would probably give this as the simplest of explanations: the Reiki practitioner brings life force energy through their hands to the recipient. This induces the relaxation response and activates and enhances the body's natural ability to heal itself. The energy goes to where it is needed most at that moment—the physical, mental, emotional or spiritual level of the person's being. It moves out blocked energies, cleanses the body of toxins, and works to create a state of balance.

Since more healthcare practitioners are becoming involved in Reiki, they have been searching for a more scientific explanation. As a holistic nurse, I particularly like the explanation of Dr. James Oschman[1] when he describes how practitioners of hands-on therapies can emit extremely low frequency (ELF) signals from their hands. These are related to the idea of magnetic fields and how they can jump start the healing process in various tissues of the body. It was also noted that this pulsing field is produced by the hands of practitioners of touch therapies but not by non-practitioners. In essence, once could say that biomagnetic fields produced by a practitioner's hand can induce current flows in the tissues and cells of individuals who are in close proximity to stimulate the repair of one or more tissues.

As a nurse and Reiki Master Teacher, I believe that when a Reiki practitioner begins giving Reiki, feelings of compassion and other healing feelings are created in their heart. These feelings can positively affect the electrical energies of their heart, which in turn travel through their nerves and vascular system into their hands. This then creates a healing biofield that can be transmitted to the recipient.

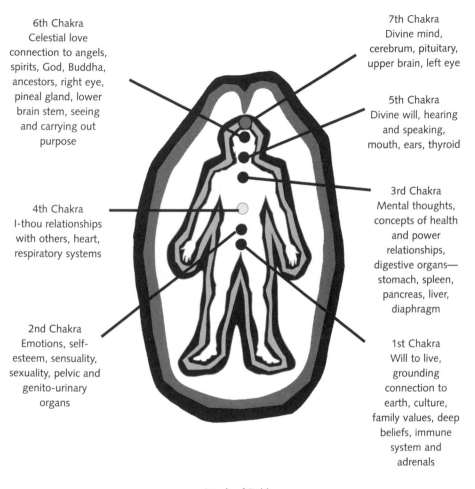

6th Chakra
Celestial love
connection to angels,
spirits, God, Buddha,
ancestors, right eye,
pineal gland, lower
brain stem, seeing
and carrying out
purpose

7th Chakra
Divine mind,
cerebrum, pituitary,
upper brain, left eye

5th Chakra
Divine will, hearing
and speaking,
mouth, ears, thyroid

4th Chakra
I-thou relationships
with others, heart,
respiratory systems

3rd Chakra
Mental thoughts,
concepts of health
and power
relationships,
digestive organs—
stomach, spleen,
pancreas, liver,
diaphragm

2nd Chakra
Emotions, self-
esteem, sensuality,
sexuality, pelvic and
genito-urinary
organs

1st Chakra
Will to live,
grounding
connection to
earth, culture,
family values, deep
beliefs, immune
system and
adrenals

Levels of Field
1. Physical (structured)
2. Emotional (unstructured)
3. Mental (structured)
4. Heart (I-thou) (unstructured)
5. Divine will (structured)
6. Divine love (unstructured)
7. Divine mind (structured)

Figure 20.1 **The Chakra Illustrated**
Source: Reprinted with permission from *Nurse Practitioner Forum*, 9: 211, Stern: "The human energy field" Copyright 1998, Elsevier, Inc.

Reiki is classified as a biofield energy technique. The charkas, or energy centers, correlate to major nerve ganglia from the spinal cord. There are seven charkas in the body.

You could also say that the heart chakra is opened wide when one feels compassion and wishes to reduce the suffering of others; that energy travels down the related meridian (energy pathway) to the palms of the hands. Thus the compassion and intent to help another opens the palm chakras and the healing energy flows. This is probably the basis of all hands-on healing, from ancient times to today.

Q: How many people use Reiki?

A: It is hard to give a number, but I would venture to say millions of people know and use Reiki. It is popular all over the world. You can go to various Reiki websites and see that they have an international directory of Reiki practitioners and teachers in Europe, India, Japan, the United States, Canada, Asia, Africa, Australia, the United Kingdom, Ireland, and Indonesia to name just a few.

Q: What research has been done?

A: Medical research on the use of Reiki is still in the infancy stages. Since Reiki is a multidimensional experience (body, mind, and spirit), measuring its effects can often be a challenge. Reiki is considered a form of life force energy, commonly referred to as chi (ki, Qi, prana, etc.). Reiki is often considered an offshoot of the practice of Qigong, where one gathers and strengthens one's chi for healing. Chen and Turner[2] describes how Traditional Chinese Medicine (TCM) postulates the existence of a subtle energy (Qi) that circulates through the body. TCM believes that when the Qi is strengthened or balanced, it can improve health and ward off or slow the progress of disease. A case study was conducted to see if the study and use of Qigong could help a man suffering from chronic conditions and multiple symptoms. They found that intensive training and daily use resulted in a simultaneous recovery from multiple incurable conditions. The authors concluded that the success could not be explained by any *known* medical theories and called for formal clinical trials to examine this self-healing energy therapy.

Englebretson and Wardell[3] reported in their study that "many linear models used in researching touch therapies are not complex enough to capture the experience of participants." Dr. Schiller,[4] chairman of the Department of Family Medicine at Beth Israel Medical Center in New York, reports that "the clinical evaluation of Reiki challenges our current standards of assessment. Clinical research in this area needs to expand our definition of outcome, to include the felt experience of the patient . . . other methods must be developed and employed."

A preliminary study conducted at the Institute of Neurological Sciences at Southern General Hospital in Glasgow, United Kingdom, found that heart rate and diastolic blood pressure decreased significantly in the Reiki treated group.[5] The authors contend that the results justify further study due to the small size of the study group and the small changes noted. For a critical review of Reiki, Miles and True[6] published a review of the history, theory, practice, and research of Reiki.

Reiki has been used in pain management for cancer patients and was found to significantly reduce pain.[7,8] Another study found that when Reiki was given to terminally ill cancer patients, they experienced a peaceful and calm passing (when death was imminent), as well as relief from pain, anxiety, difficulty in breathing, and edema (swelling).[9] Shore[10] reported statistically significant decreases in symptoms of depression and stress with long term effects using Reiki. Other studies found that Reiki promoted wound healing, induced the relaxation response, decreased blood pressure, improved immune system function, and improved overall feelings of well-being. HIV patients have decreased pain and anxiety after Reiki treatments.[11]

Various hospitals are conducting their own studies of the efficacy of Reiki. George Washington University Hospital in Washington, DC, had a six month pilot program from December 2003 to June 2004 where Reiki was given before patients underwent a cardiac catheterization procedure. Although the response group was small, the report on the program noted self-reported benefits such as increased confidence and reduced anxiety.

Q: How much does a Reiki session cost?

A: The cost of a Reiki session varies. It can range from $25 to $125, based on location. Many people charge what the people in their area charge for a one hour massage. There are some people that do not charge for a Reiki session. They believe it is part of their spiritual practice and consider it being of service.

Q: Does insurance reimburse you for it?

A: There have been some companies that have reimbursed for a Reiki session but it is usually a case-by-case situation. Some insurance companies do reimburse for complementary therapies. Some people have a rider on their policy that covers complementary therapies. It is important to check with their employer or insurance company regarding insurance reimbursement. There was an insurance company in the Northeast that did reimburse for regular Reiki treatments for a teenage girl who had multiple emergency room admissions for diabetic ketoacidosis. Their payments were based on the findings that Reiki sessions helped her to maintain her blood glucose levels at a more normal range. It also decreased her ER visits.

Q: Are there any side effects or consequences to my health?

A: In 13 years of practicing Reiki, I have heard of none. Reiki is generally accepted as a low-risk modality. Reiki induces the relaxation response and all its benefits. Because Reiki balances one's energy, some people have, on occasion, experienced a temporary increase in their symptoms, that is, they feel worse before they feel better. When it does happen, the person usually feels better within 24 hours. In fact, the person usually reports that they feel more than 100% better than before the session. Perhaps it can be considered a release of toxins or balancing what is out of balance.

Q: How do I know if it is working and not something else I might be doing?

A: No one can ever be 100% sure of anything. It is hard to rule out all the variables. But if it produces results that you have never experienced before, or it happens quicker than expected, I would have to say that it is most probably Reiki. Reiki speeds up or enhances the body's natural ability to heal itself. You could also not try any other treatment or modality but Reiki to see if it is the Reiki or something else.

There are many ways to know if Reiki is helping you. If you received Reiki to prepare for surgery, you might find that your recovery time was decreased, you needed minimal pain medication, or you were up and walking about that same night. Or, your doctor might tell you that you lost less blood than people often do during that particular operation. Your doctor might tell you that you are healing quicker than expected.

If you are taking pain medication, you might find you need less. You might find that pain is gone. You might feel energized and peaceful. You might feel that your life is flowing better.

If you feel generally more relaxed, peaceful, or calm, then it is working. When the outcome is better or easier than expected, it is often Reiki.

Q: What will my doctor think about this?

A: Many doctors today are open to Reiki. Much is how it is presented or explained. If you present Reiki as a simple relaxation or energy balancing technique, many doctors are open to it. If you get into a metaphysical or "woo-woo" explanation, a doctor would probably be turned off.

Many people are requesting that their Reiki practitioner be present in the operating room during surgery. When a patient requests it, doctors often oblige. Some doctors tell their patients that are receiving Reiki, "what ever you are doing keep it up." There are many doctors that have taken Reiki classes as well.

Dr. Schiller[4] states that with "self-treatment, simple techniques, and the use of energy and spirit, Reiki introduces the practitioner to essential elements of Integrative Medicine and its ability to make even the most conventionally oriented physician more effective and compassionate." So I think a lot more doctors are open to Reiki than we think.

Q: Do I need to approve Reiki with my doctor before I start using it?

A: No. Reiki does no harm. It is, at its simplest, a relaxation technique. It relaxes body, mind, and spirit. Thus it is often a multisensory experience.

Q: Does Reiki interact with any medications I am taking?

A: Not that I am aware of. I know several nurse anesthetists and doctors that give Reiki as they are giving anesthesia. They tell me that the patient is usually more relaxed, needs less anesthesia, and has an easier time coming out of the anesthesia. Some people that have received Reiki during radiation treatment or chemotherapy have told me they had less nausea and recovered quicker.

Q: Should regular pain medications be discontinued when doing Reiki?

A: Reiki does not take the place of medication and should not be used for such. However, because of its relaxation effects and overall benefits, some people have found that they might require less medication. All medication adjustments should be done under the supervision of a doctor.

Q: Does one have to be certified or licensed in Reiki?

A: No, there is no one licensing or certifying agency for Reiki. There are different schools and philosophies about Reiki so it would be difficult to set standards for all. However, some states are lobbying to have Reiki practitioners obtain a massage license so they can regulate its practice. Please note: *Reiki is not a form of massage.* Many states are working to keep Reiki and other complementary healing methods free of government regulation. California has the health freedom act (**www.californiahealthfreedom.org/ documents/our_bill.asp***) and a bill is now in the New York senate to make Reiki a legal practice without the need of a government issued license (**www.NYNaturalhealthproject.org**).

One can start doing Reiki as soon as they take their first class. My youngest son was four years old when I taught him Reiki. It is simply turning on or awakening a person's ability to bring in healing energy. Having the intention to help someone gets it started. Bringing in and working with life force energy is a natural ability that we all have. It requires only the intention to help or heal.

Q: How is Reiki different than other hands-on healing modalities?

A: The Reiki attunement is what makes Reiki different from other hands-on healing techniques. The attunement is an empowerment or energy balancing technique that the Master Teacher does for each student. The attunement balances a person's energy and helps them to be open to bring in and hold this life force energy. Everyone is born with the ability to bring in universal life force energy. Reiki is one way to turn on or work with this life force energy.

Q: How does one learn Reiki? What kind of training is there?

A: Learning Reiki is very easy. You simply attend a Reiki workshop, receive an attunement (energy balancing technique), learn the basic hands-on positions, and one can begin.

In its simplest form, Reiki is a hands-on healing technique that induces relaxation, decreases stress, and also promotes healing. It is that easy. Reiki develops from committed practice. Of note is the fact that because of the empowerment or attunement, Reiki cannot be learned from a book.

There are different schools or approaches to learning and doing Reiki. The person usually finds the teacher and learning method that works best for them. Most Reiki training is divided into levels: Reiki I, Reiki II, Advanced Reiki, and Master Teacher (see **Table 20.1**).

Table 20.1   Training Levels for Reiki

Reiki Levels	Description
Reiki I (one or two days of training)	• the history of Reiki and the Reiki Ideals • what it is and how it heals • the attunement • the hand positions for giving and receiving • Reiki hands-on practice
Reiki II (usually a one day class)	• learning the Reiki symbols (tools to enhance the flow of Reiki) • the Reiki II attunement • how to send Reiki at a distance • hands-on practice
Advanced Reiki (usually a one or two day workshop)	• advanced symbols • chakra balancing or other techniques • the advanced attunement • aura balancing techniques • moving meditations (like a tai chi or Qigong exercise)
Reiki Master Teacher (done by attending a weekend workshop or a mentoring program of 6 months to a year)	• the Master attunement • healing attunement • meditation to increase the flow of chi throughout the body • master symbols • values and ethics • learning how to give all levels of attunements

Some schools require a mentorship or apprenticeship to become a Master Teacher. That may include a required number of hours of practice or number of sessions, working with a mentor, co-teaching classes, starting and leading a Reiki Circle, doing presentations on Reiki, or learning how to conduct oneself as a professional (ethics, teaching and learning, business aspects, dynamics of the healing relationship, etc.). Once again it is important to remember that Reiki plain and simple is putting one's hands on a person to bring in healing energy. That is why it is so easy to learn and so easy to teach.

Q: Can anyone do Reiki?

A: Yes, it is simply the intent to help or heal that gets it started. Anyone with an open and caring heart can do Reiki. As I said earlier, my youngest son was four years old when I taught him Reiki.

Q: Is Reiki being used in hospitals and other health facilities? In what capacity?

A: Reiki is becoming more and more widely used in hospitals all over the world. One reason is that hospitals are more receptive to CAMs to maintain a competitive edge in marketing to patients as consumers. Others want to maintain or improve patient care.

There are many hospitals that now offer Reiki as part of their patient services. Dartmouth Hitchcock Medical Center, NH; Integrative Medicine Outpatient Center at Memorial Sloan Kettering Cancer Center, NY; Integrative Therapies Program for Children with Cancer at Columbia Presbyterian Medical Center, NY, all offer Reiki for their patients with cancer.

Jackson describes how at Memorial Sloan Kettering Cancer Center in New York City, Reiki is offered to improve the quality of life and help relieve the symptoms of cancer. They found that Reiki helps to eliminate pain and stress which leaves more energy for the body to heal itself.

Reiki is also offered at Mercy Hospital, ME; Center for Integrative Medicine at George Washington University Hospital, Washington, DC; Samuels Center for Comprehensive Care at St. Lukes-Roosevelt Hospital Center, NY; Tucson Medical Center, AZ; California Pacific Medical Center, CA; Portsmouth Regional Hospital, NH; Marin General Hospital, CA; University of Michigan Hospital, MI; The Manhattan Eye, Ear, and Throat Hospital, NY; Virginia Hospital, Arlington, VA; North Shore Medical Center (NSMC) Women's Center, Danvers, MA; NSMC Cancer Center, Peabody, MA, as well as many others.

Reiki is being used in hospices, rehabilitation facilities, detoxification units, HIV/AIDs facilities or clinics, nursing homes, and children's hospitals, to name but a few. Brownes Cancer Support Clinic in Perth, Australia, sees 300 patients with cancer every month for Reiki sessions.

As recipients of a grant, The Coventry Community Drug Team in the United Kingdom integrates Reiki with counseling and stress management in their substance abuse program with much success. They have found that Reiki brings deep relaxation of body and mind and allows the participant to reach deeper levels of healing. Other detoxification and recovery programs have reported similar benefits.

Reiki is being used in various capacities in healthcare facilities. Some have it as part of their preparation and recovery from surgery. Reiki practitioners are often allowed in the operating room (per patient request and permission of surgeon) to give Reiki during surgery. Nurses that do Reiki give it to the patients within their nursing practice. People are receiving Reiki before and after radiation or chemotherapy treatments, in the Recovery Room, during labor and delivery, in the emergency room, during diagnostic procedures or in preparation for, and even at staff meetings.

Some hospitals have volunteers that give Reiki to patients in their rooms. Staff that has been trained in Reiki often give it to their fellow workers in times of stress or simply as part of their everyday work. Other hospitals have Reiki Circles or shares that are run by nurses and/or Reiki practitioners. These can be attended by anyone who wishes to receive Reiki.

Giving Reiki is also about a healthcare provider simply touching a person or holding their hand and allowing the life force energy to flow through them to the person. Reiki can be given this simply. It is a compassionate and caring touch. Even five minutes of Reiki is like receiving a boost of energy or a calming influence. One of the reasons Reiki has become so popular with healthcare professionals is that it helps them to reconnect with the essence of true healing: compassion and unconditional regard.

Suggested Reading

Barnett L, Chambers M. *Reiki Energy Medicine*. Rochester, VT: Healing Arts Press; 1996.

Benor D. *Spiritual Healing: Scientific Validation of a Healing Revolution*. Southfield, MI: Vision Publications; 2002.

Goldner D. *Infinite Grace: Where the Worlds of Science and Spiritual Healing Meet*. Charlottesville, VA: Hampton Roads; 1999.

Honervogt T, *The Power of Reiki*. New York, NY: Henry Holt and Co; 1998.

Lubeck W, Rand W, Petter FA. *The Spirit of Reiki*. Twin Lakes, WI: Lotus Press; 2001.

Rand W. *Reiki: The Healing Touch*. Southfield, MI: Vision Publication; 1996.

Reiki News Magazine. Available at: www.reiki.org

International Center for Reiki Training. Available at: www.reiki.org

Reiki Medical Info/Research. Available at www.reikimedresearch.com

International Association of Reiki Professionals. Available at: www.iarp.org

James Oschman. Available at www.energyresearch.bizland.com

Pamela Miles. Available at: www.pamelamiles.com

References

1. Oschman J. *Energy Medicine: The Scientific Basis*. London: Churchill Livingston; 2000.
2. Chen K, Turner F. A case study of simultaneous recovery from multiple physical symptoms with medical Qigong therapy. *J Altern Complement Med*. 2004;10(1):159–162.
3. Engebretson J, Wardell D. Experience of a reiki session. *Altern Ther Health Med*. 2002;8(2):48–53.
4. Schiller R. Reiki: a starting point for integrative medicine. *Altern Ther Health Med*. 2003;9(2):20–21.
5. Mackay N, Hansen S, McFarlane, O. Autonomic nervous system changes during reiki treatment: a preliminary study. *J Altern Complement Med*. 2004;10(6):1077–1081.
6. Miles P, True G. Reiki—review of a biofield therapy: history, theory, practice and research. *Altern Ther Health Med*. 2003;9(2)62–72.
7. Olson K, Hanson J. Using Reiki to manage painL: a preliminary report. *Cancer Prev Control*. 1997;1(2):108–113.
8. Olson K, Hanson J, Michaud M. A phase II trial for Reiki for the management of pain in advanced cnacer patients. J Pain Symptom Manage. 2003;26(5):990–997.
9. Bullock M. Reiki: a complementary therapy for life. *Am J Hosp Palliat Care*. 1997;14(1):31–33.
10. Shore A. Long-term effects of energetic healing on symptoms of psychological depression and self-perceived stress. *Altern Therap Health Med*. 2004;10(3):42–48.
11. Miles P. Preliminary report on the use of Reiki HIV-related pain and anxiety. *Altern Ther Health Med*. 2003;9(2):36.
12. Jackson K. Reiki: rising star in complementary cancer care. *Radiology Today*. 2003;4(10):9–13.

21

Therapeutic Touch

Patricia Smyth, DSN, RN, FNP-C

About the Author

Patricia Smyth is a family nurse practitioner and director of the graduate nursing program at Western Carolina University. She has had an interest in Therapeutic Touch (TT) since 1976 when Delores Kreiger presented a day long seminar on TT at a hospital where she was employed as a new nurse. Dr. Smyth has done research with TT and pediatrics and incorporates TT in the care of her patients.

Q: What is Therapeutic Touch (TT)?

A: Therapeutic Touch is a healing intervention that was started by a nurse, Delores Kreiger. Back in the 1960s and 1970s, Kreiger observed healers using their hands to make people feel better. One of these healers was Dorothy Kunz. Kreiger worked with Kunz to learn the technique. Kreiger named the technique Therapeutic Touch (TT). Kreiger believed that people are made of energy fields that can be altered for the better with the use of the TT practitioner's hands moving just above the skin. She started teaching other nurses how to use this technique. Over the intervening years, many nurses and interested people have learned to provide this intervention. When a person is feeling unwell, either physically or mentally, blocks occur in their energy field. These blocks prevent the person from improving their health. In other words, the block prevents energy from moving smoothly. A TT practitioner evaluates what is happening with the individual and then reshapes and unblocks the energy field of the person. The goal of TT is to attain a smooth, stable energy state in which the person can heal himself or herself.

Q: How did you get interested in TT?

A: The hospital where I worked had a nursing seminar where Delores Kreiger came to speak and demonstrate. The participants treated each other as a way to practice. Initially I thought it was all mumbo-jumbo, however I started treating some of my patients with amazing success and I was hooked! The first time I used TT in practice was with a little 6-week-old girl who had just had surgery to repair a cleft lip. She was crying inconsolably and her parents were upset because they could not comfort her. The physician commented that crying would place a stress on the stitches. I picked her up and with her parent's permission did TT for about 5 minutes. Much to their amazement, she quieted and went to sleep. I use TT almost daily in my practice when I can get the patient's or parent's permission. When I moved from bedside nursing to teaching, I included TT in my lectures through demonstrations and supervised students who performed the technique on patients. The students really love the idea that this is an independent nursing intervention they can provide for their patients.

Q: How does TT work?

A: As I mentioned before, TT works on the person's energy system; some may understand it better if I say a force field. Just as you have electrocardiogram or brain wave patterns, TT practitioners believe that the whole body is made up with a pattern of energy. Have you ever met a person that you felt had good vibes? Well these vibes can get out of pattern or blocked so the person is not able to use their own energy effectively. What the TT practitioner does is

- slowly assess what the pattern feels like for the patient, going from the head to the toe noting areas of heat, coldness, or heaviness;

- use short movements 1 to 3 inches over the body, shaking the practitioners hands to remove any heavy feelings;
- use the hands to remove the blockages that have occurred; and
- smooth the hands in long sweeping movements to make the individual feel better and assure all areas have been addressed.

Our ability to cope with healing is much better after receiving treatment. Healing, as a term, does not necessarily mean a "cure"; rather it can be dissimilar effects for people related to their specific needs. The person may feel better, sleep better, or perhaps initially may feel no different. Some people report feeling more relaxed. It will not cure any disease state but will enable the recipient to handle their recovery more effectively.

Q: Why do you believe in TT?

A: I believe in TT because I've seen it work. Even I was skeptical when I took my first seminar. At first I thought that this was just a new age approach that had no basis in reality, but I became a believer when I saw the powerful outcomes despite my non-believer status. It is hard to argue with success. Countless times I treated dyed-in-the-wool skeptics who turned out to be my greatest supporters. I do believe that some people have an innate gift to share, but I really do conclude that most individuals have the capability to become TT practitioners if they are able to center themselves. Centering is a means of concentration that is absolute, focusing only on the recipient. Providing TT *does* take concentration. I truly love providing TT, and as an interesting side note, it makes me feel better too!

Q: What conditions respond to TT treatment?

A: I have personally used TT for a variety of symptoms including: HIV/AIDS; headaches or body aches; prior to child immunizations (who reported less pain following the injection); cancer patients, not as a cure, but simply to improve their quality of life; prior to chemotherapy to prevent nausea and vomiting; pre- and post-operative pain control; addiction disorders; anxiety; fibromyalgia; grief from loss of a spouse/parent/child; and orthopedic injuries.

All of the conditions listed here have responded very well to TT. There are many other conditions that respond well to TT, such as muscle strain, arthritis, minor injuries, respiratory conditions, neurological illnesses, gastrointestinal conditions, and many others.

Q: Can there be negative outcomes for my health using TT?

A: In all the years I have used TT, I have had no negative outcomes from using this modality. There have been no accounts in the literature except when a nurse tried to use TT as the *only* treatment for postoperative pain. Therapeutic Touch should be considered as something to use in addition to medication, not in place of medication. I would never encourage any one to avoid standard therapy, but I do encourage the use of TT as a complement to standard care. The nurses from whom I learned the technique cautioned the use of TT with pregnant women because the effects for the fetus are unknown, however, no study has been identified that suggests negative outcomes for any fetus thus far. Practitioners recommend that caution should be used in the area of the head. I have discovered that when patients have headaches and I use TT around the head and neck area, all the recipients experience relief with no negative outcomes to their health.

Q: How is TT done?

A: To start with, the practitioner must have consent from the person being treated. If the person is unable to ask for the treatment, a family member may request it for a loved one who may not be able to consent (e.g., a child or someone postoperatively). The practitioner will do TT by making the person comfortable, either by sitting or lying. I like to use a massage table, but all practitioners vary in their preferences. The practitioner will take a moment to prepare; this is called centering. The practitioner will use their hands, palms down, 1 to 3 inches above the body, starting at the head and finishing at the feet. Once the practitioner assesses the person, they will then start providing the treatment using sweeping motions to mobilize the energy field and smooth out blockages. The practitioner will shake their hands when they feel heavy. Krieger called this unruffling. Areas identified by the practitioner as blocked are worked on more than other areas. The practitioner will then complete an overall sweep of the body to check for continued blockages. The treatment will be completed once the energy field feels smooth. The session may be as short as 5 minutes or as long as 30 minutes, depending on the person's need for treatment and their response to treatment. Some patients may only require one or two sessions. Generally the more chronic the problem, the more sessions are required to help the recipient.

Q: What will I feel during a session?

A: While responses vary, many people report a feeling of warmth over the areas the practitioner is working. Some individuals report a tingling sensation, others report total relaxation. Many of my clients actually fall asleep during treatment. I have had many clients report no changes at the time, however, they later tell me that they slept better and had a decrease in the symptoms for which they sought treatment. One child, who had been having TT to treat his arm in a cast, actually was able to have the cast off much earlier than expected. But please understand, this could just be happenstance.

Q: About how much does TT cost per session?

A: Treatment with TT varies from $20 to $90 per session. Some practitioners will do a group of sessions for a lower price. For example, three sessions may cost $120, rather than $50 per session, because it may take several sessions initially to achieve maximum relief. When a person is unfamiliar with how the technique is done, they are not as relaxed; therefore, it may take a couple of treatments.

Q: Can I wear my regular clothes for a session?

A: You can wear regular clothes for a session. I do recommend that any metal such as belt buckles or watches, are removed prior to treatment. Otherwise any light clothing is perfectly fine. I really prefer that my clients wear more natural fabrics such as cotton or wool. I do recommend that the person choose clothing they will be most comfortable in lying down.

Q: Are their any contraindications to using TT?

A: There are no documented contraindications using TT. However, I have observed through my practice that children appear to respond more rapidly to TT. I recommend that those treating pregnant women for longer than 15 minutes could possibly be too intense for the fetus. If a child or an adult starts getting restless, it is a signal to cease the treatment. No studies have ever been conducted to answer this concern. I suggest that research, perhaps conducting a TT session while a woman was receiving fetal monitoring, could potentially provide some answers to guide our practice.

Q: Should I tell my healthcare provider I want to try TT?

A: As always, it is important to consult with your healthcare provider for any use of complementary or alternative interventions. Some providers may dismiss the treatment; however, more providers are now aware that these methods have positive outcomes. I have had patients referred to me by physicians and nurse practitioners for treatment.

Q: Are there any interactions with my medications with TT?

A: Because TT is a mechanism that interacts with your energy field, no interactions are seen with medications. However, individuals who take antihypertensive agents will need to use extra precautions when arising from the massage table because their blood pressure is decreased due to total body relaxation. These individuals should sit up first and get their bearings before standing.

Q: Have you treated many people?

A: I have been practicing TT for around 30 years so you can imagine how many individuals I have treated. I would be unable to provide you with a guess but I can safely say hundreds.

Q: Can you give me some examples how TT works?

A: I have provided a few examples, but I have some more interesting ones. I cared for a young man in a hospital who had been in an automobile accident two days before. He had been in intensive care and just got transferred to the regular floor. He was in traction to hold his broken leg in alignment. He was crying in pain when I came on duty. He had received his pain medication an hour and a half ago, but was still experiencing pain. I did readjust his position, thinking that perhaps misalignment was the cause of his pain, and put in a call to the doctor. In the meantime, I asked him if he wanted me to do TT. After I explained what TT was he said OK, but he was very skeptical. I started his treatment and had been working with him for about 7 minutes when he started dozing off. His doctor came into the room at this point and just stood there watching. After I concluded the treatment (the patient was still sleeping) I went out of the room to discuss his case with the doctor. She asked what I had been doing to the patient and was pleased when I explained about TT. She said that she really hadn't wanted to increase his pain medication and perhaps she didn't need to now that he was asleep. Despite my success, I did convince her to increase his medication, explaining that TT was an adjunct to medication, not a replacement for it. I treated this young man one more time before I went off duty and gave him his increased dose. He slept through the night and had a rapid recovery from his injuries.

Another instance that stands out in my mind is when I was researching how preschool children responded to receiving TT prior to their immunizations. I needed to obtain consent from the caregivers to treat the children. One of the young boys who ended up in the TT treatment group appeared very frightened about getting his immunizations. His mother explained that he had asthma and had been hospitalized on many occasions. While he was in the hospital he had to be strongly restrained in order to receive intravenous therapy, have blood drawn, or have any procedures done. His mother said, right in front of the child, that he wasn't going to hold still for his shots and we were wasting our time doing anything but holding him down. I thought at the time, "Oh no! She just told him to misbehave!" I started his TT treatment and he watched me closely for a couple of minutes, then he relaxed visibly. By the time I stopped his treatment he was nearly asleep. He never moved for his immunizations, never cried, and reported that he really didn't feel the shots. I was amazed and his mother was astonished! She told me she wanted me around for his next hospitalization.

I also provided TT for a 45-year-old man who was planning to have surgery for metastatic colon cancer. The doctor told him his cancer was "about the size of a fist" very close to the rectal opening, and he had several lesions on his liver. I treated the patient two times a week for three weeks. He went into the hospital and had the surgery. The surgeon reported that when he went in, he couldn't find the original cancer despite having performed an endoscope on the patient just a week before I started the treatment. While my providing the patient with TT did not remove the cancer, I did work with his own energy field to allow him to heal that particular site. This was four years ago. The patient has had chemotherapy and thus far has not succumbed to the cancer. He has worked full time and receives TT on a weekly or as needed basis. He feels that the chemotherapy and TT have been the winning combination in his battle to live.

Sometimes peers can be the biggest critics. I was working one day and had just provided TT to one of my patients when one of the nurses said she had a bad headache. She was about to go home for her medicine when she challenged me to get rid of her headache. I hated to be put on the spot but I could tell she really was in pain. I told her that I would treat her but she was to go home regardless. I treated her for about 15 minutes. She reported that the headache was less intense so she felt safer driving. When she got home she called me and said her headache was totally gone. It had disappeared while driving home. She never did take her medicine.

Q: What school did you attend to learn about TT?

A: I attended an 8 hour workshop at the hospital where I worked and sought out several other TT seminars afterwards. One seminar was from Binghamton University and the other from the Holistic Nurses Association. When I went to graduate school at the University of Alabama at Birmingham for my doctorate in nursing, I took a course in TT that was a springboard for my dissertation.

Q: Have you conducted any research in TT?

A: Yes, I conducted a study called "Immunization Pain Perception in Preschool Children Using Therapeutic Touch."[1] I had three groups of parent-child participants. The children were placed randomly in one of three groups. One group simply had an observer, one group had their hands held by a research assistant, and one group received TT from me. The outcome of the study indicated that the TT group had the lowest pain level. The parents reported the childs' behavior as indicating less distress in the TT group. The parents also reported greater satisfaction with care in the TT group. I also published an article discussing a case where I provided TT both pre- and postoperatively for a 64-year-old man with cancer of the pancreas. In the article I discuss the advantages of providing both standard care and TT for an improved outcome for the patient. This gentleman has since died but his wife strongly believes that he did not have pain because he received TT on a weekly or twice weekly basis. He actually died from a heart attack brought on by a blood clot and not from his cancer.[2]

Q: How many years does it take to learn this technique?

A: To be quite honest, I have taught students to do TT in three classes and they have been good beginners at the end of the course. If a person has the ability, they very quickly pick it up. It is very important to practice on a daily or at least weekly basis to remain competent in the skill. That takes commitment and dedication. One student had only one demonstration class when her father had a heart attack. She used TT on him in the hospital and his blood pressure and pulse rate stabilized. He had surgery and she provided him with TT every night. He was out of intensive care in 10 hours following bypass surgery and out of the hospital in three days. She was committed to her father's improvement and was able to maintain her concentration toward that goal.

Q: Does insurance reimburse for TT?

A: Insurance does not reimburse in most cases. Of the patients who were referred by physicians, only one was reimbursed in all the time I have been providing TT treatments. I can tell you that I have not quit my day job to do this work either.

Q: Are you certified or licensed in TT?

A: I have three certificates from completing TT courses but this was only for continuing education credits, not by a credential providing organization. I did receive college credits for a university course. There is a Nurse Healers-Professional Associates International, Inc., organization where you can become recognized as a Therapeutic Touch teacher for $700. This was not available when I first started with TT and at this point I do not regard this recognition as imperative.

Suggested Readings

Nurse Healer's Professional Association International. Available at: www.therapeutic-touch.org

Therapeutic Touch. Available at: www.therapeutictouch.com.

Pumpkin Hollow Farm available at: http://www.pumpkinhollow.org/tt.html.

Krieger D. *Therapeutic Touch: How To Use Your Hands To Heal.* Englewood Cliffts, NJ: Prentice Hall; 1979.

Krieger D. *Accepting Your Power To Heal: The Personal Practice of Therapeutic Touch.* Santa Fe, NM: Bear & Co; 1993.

Krieger, D. *Therapeutic Touch: Inner Workbook.* Santa Fe, NM: Bear & Co; 1997.

Macrae, J. (1998) *Therapeutic Touch: Practical Techniques for Healing through the Vitl-Energy Field,* True Sounds, co. Audio Cassette. New York: Alfred A. Knopf; 1998.

References

1. Smyth PE. Reducing immuniztion pain perception in preschoolers with therapeutic touch. [Doctoral Disseration, Research] (The University of Alabama at Birmingham), 1999; D.S.N. 119p AN:20005062852.

2. Smyth PE. Therapeutic touch for a patient after a Whipple procedure. *Crit Care Nurs Clin North Am.* 2001;13(3):357–363.

22

Bioelectromagnetic Therapy

Norma G. Cuellar, DSN, RN, CCRN

About the Author

Norma G. Cuellar is a registered nurse who has a doctoral degree in adult health nursing. She was an independent consultant for magnetic therapy before she decided to pursue a research career in Complementary and Alternative Medicine. She did a one year post-doctoral fellowship in Complementary and Alternative Medicine at the University of Virginia. She currently is an assistant professor at the University of Pennsylvania School of Nursing where she does research in a variety of areas related to Complementary and Alternative Medicine.

Q: What got you interested in bioelectromagnetic therapy?

A: As a nurse educator, I had a former student come to my office to chat. I asked what he was doing and he told me he had his own business working with magnets. I thought he was crazy! I had some chronic low back pain that I had just tolerated for many years, assuming it was part of the aging process. He asked me if I wanted to try some of the magnet. I slept on a sleep pad and used some products for my back. Within the first week, my back discomfort was gone and I was sleeping like a baby, something I had not done in many years.

Q: Are their different types of magnetic therapy?

A: Yes, there are. For the purpose of this chapter, I will refer to bioelectromagnetic therapy as magnets or magnetic therapy. There are many different types of magnetic therapy but essentially you have two classifications in relation to treatment: permanent or static magnets and electromagnets.

Permanent magnets are those used in alternative therapies and are purchased at a variety of retail stores or on the Internet. These magnets are not dependent upon electrical current and are constantly giving off magnetic energy because of their molecular makeup and processing. They are easy to use, readily available when needed, and cheaper than electromagnets. They come in a variety of forms: insoles, wraps, bracelets, necklaces, metallic pieces to put on body, seats, mattresses, pillows, and sleep masks.

Electromagnets are produced through an electrical current that can be turned on and off, are always in motion, and are stronger than permanent magnets. These magnets are regulated by the Food and Drug Administration (FDA) and are found in hospitals or healthcare agencies. They are not mobile. The patient goes in for a treatment that is in a controlled environment with an intervention that is measurable by dose, time, and frequency.

Q: Why do you believe in magnetic therapy?

A: I was not easily convinced when I began to use my magnets. I did a lot of reading and studying. As an educator and researcher, I immediately looked for scientific evidence to prove that these worked. The more I read and learned, the more I realized this could be plausible. I found research studies that did show significance in placebo and treatment groups using magnets.

I also began working with people who had conditions that had not been treated successfully with conventional medicine. I saw some "miracles" with people who used these products and was impressed with how they worked and their effectiveness. I published a case study that describes the benefits of magnets in a woman with rheumatoid arthritis.[1]

Q: Does magentic therapy really work?

A: I am a believer. Yes, they work, but they don't work all the time and they don't work on every health condition. I find that about 75–80% of the time, people got relief from the conditions they complain about or begin to feel better. There are usually three reasons why a magnet does not work.

1. It was not used properly (instructions are not often given when products are purchased).
2. It was not used for long enough time (one week of continuous use).
3. The dose of the magnet was not high enough. The dose of a magnet is measured in units of gauss much like a light bulb's output is measured in units of watts. Gauss represents the number of north and south poles in one square centimeter of magnet. A refrigerator magnet has about 100 gauss; a variety of magnets worn on the body have from 500–2000 gauss; an electromagnetic medical device has 20,000 gauss; and an MRI has approximately 30,000 gauss. The size of a magnet does not indicate its strength. Magnetic strength depends on the coercivity of the magnet's makeup. The horseshoe magnet is an example of a magnet with high coercivity; it has increased magnetic strength because of its specific design and shape.

Q: How do magnets work?

A: This is a very good question. No one really knows how magnets work on the body. We do know that the human body is complex with electrochemical processes that are not clearly understood. Magnetite, a strongly magnetic mineral, has been found in the human brain, heart, lung, and spleen tissue raising speculation that magnetite may have some biological function. This may support some of the theories being studied to determine the effects of magnets on the human body, including increased blood flow; increased energy through the body's meridian systems; stimulation of electrical impulses in the nervous system; direct effect on the pineal gland; realignment of certain molecules in the membranes of the cells; inhibition of the build-up of cholinesterase (an enzyme found in nerve endings that inactivates acetylcholine, which is essential in pain control); reduction of acid build-up in the body; and the Hall Effect—charged ions become more active when they pass through a magnetic field causing heat, dilatation of blood vessels, better oxygenation of tissues, and an increased ability of cells to eliminate toxins.

Magnets are applied directly on the body, usually over an area of discomfort. Each individual responds differently to the use of magnets. Often a person can feel the magnet immediately, which is described as a sensation of increased warmth or tingling. Some people get immediate relief from their discomfort; others get results within 7–10 days. Permanent magnets should be worn consistently as health outcomes improve over an extended period of time.

Q: How many people use magnets?

A: While it is unknown how many people use magnets, it is estimated that people are spending $5 billion dollars on magnets worldwide, with $5 million from the United States.[2] Eighteen percent of persons with rheumatoid arthritis, osteoarthritis, and fibromyalgia use magnets—the second most used CAM for this cohort.[3] Many people do not report that they use magnets because of embarrassment or fear of being ridiculed. Another attribute to the uncertainty of how many people use magnets is that they can be purchased in a variety of settings including the Internet, drug stores, retail stores, furniture stores, and jewelry stores to name a few. There is hardly a place where you can not buy magnets.

Q: What are magnets used for?

A: While magnets are not FDA approved medical devices, we cannot say magnets cure anything. However, people with the following conditions have found some benefit in the use of magnets:

- Allergic reactions
- Arthritis
- Chronic fatigue syndrome
- Depression
- Diabetic angiopathies
- Fibromyalgia
- Head injuries
- Inflammatory diseases
- Migraine headaches
- Menstrual pain
- Multiple Sclerosis
- Pain (immediate, acute, and chronic)
- Parkinson's disease
- Placental insufficiency
- Polio
- Respiratory problems
- Sinusitis
- Tourette's Syndrome
- Trophic ulcers
- Urinary problems
- Vascular problems
- Whiplash
- Wound healing

Q: What are safety issues related to magnets?

A: Persons who have pacemakers should check with their physician to determine safety issues. It is usually discouraged to use magnetic products anywhere around a pacemaker.

Generally, they are very safe. There has never been a reported death of someone who used magnets. Some people may have exacerbation of symptoms after beginning to use magnets, much like the first week that you begin an exercise program and have soreness. The use of magnets should not take the place of good, sensible health practices, like sound nutrition and proper exercise. Standard, conventional medical treatment should not be ignored.

Q: What type of research has been done?

A: A large amount of research has been done on magnetic therapies in the European and Eastern communities. Findings from the studies are conflicting. Much of the research in the United States has been in the use of electromagnets and has yielded more consistent results. These electromagnets are considered medical devices and provide more consistent results due to the rigor or intervention of these studies which 1) are conducted in a more controlled environment (hospitals and healthcare agencies), 2) use a controlled treatment (devices give off an exact amount of energy for an exact amount of time), 3) use an experimental design (control group and experimental group is accessible), and 4) have specific measurable outcomes.

Many critics of magnetic therapy say that it is a placebo effect that causes improved outcomes. This has been a continuing problem in the area of research, as sham products are often easy to make. It is a very challenging area of research that presents many questions related to methodology and design. The National Center for Complementary and Alternative Medicine now has a web site specifically for information on research and magnets available at **http://nccam.nih.gov/health/magnet/magnet.htm**.

Q: How much does it cost?

A: The cost varies. It is important to take note that you pay for what you get. The quality of the magnetic products that you purchase is not always the same. You can purchase some products for as low as $5 with bed pads and blankets and accessories up to thousands of dollars.

Q: Does insurance reimburse you for it?

A: Actually, some insurance have reimbursed depending on how the product is being used and how it is coded. If it is used for supportive products or splints, for example, some insurances may reimburse you for it.

Q: Are there any consequences to my health?

A: No, you can discontinue the use of a magnetic product as quickly as you can take it on or off. The only concern will be if you have a pacemaker.

Q: How do I know if it is working and not something else I am doing?

A: This is a difficult question. Some people will feel an immediate sensation when the magnet is applied to their body, like tingling, itching, or warmth. This is a sign that something is going on! Persons who use magnets may find that they don't have to take as many pain medications. I know of one person who was paying over $500 per month in prescription medications. After three months of using magnets, her pharmacy bill was down to $150. The only thing she had changed was the use of magnets. Many people use themselves as their own control. They use the product for an extended period of time and then take it off and see if there is a difference. If the symptoms come back, chances are the magnets were working.

Q: What will my doctor think about this?

A: I think more doctors are becoming aware of the popularity of the use of Complementary and Alternative Medicine (CAM). With recent studies that show patients are reluctant to even talk to their doctors about CAM use, physicians are not as verbal in their opposition in the use of alternative products. It really depends on who your doctor is and what he believes about CAM. I can tell you now, most people think magnets are quackery and think it is crazy. It is up to you to decide what is best for you and your own health care.

Q: Do I need to approve magnetic therapy with my doctor before I start using it?

A: This is a question that you must answer. If a complementary or alternative therapy is ingested, it may have interactions with other medications that could be significant, and I would say yes, let the doctor know you are taking the herb or natural product. Magnets do not fall in this category. If you have worse discomfort after you begin to use the magnets and go to the doctor, you should tell him that you are using magnets. I would discontinue the magnets first.

I had one lady who had discomfort in her stomach. She said the discomfort was not continuous. She wanted to use something to help with the discomfort without taking narcotics. She decided to use the magnets to see if it would help. When she began using the magnets, her discomfort worsened. I told her to stop using the magnets and go to the doctor. She was diagnosed with gall bladder disease and had surgery. I hear stories like this frequently and often think that the magnets, while they may not have alleviated the discomfort, exacerbated another health condition that needed to be treated.

Q: Will this hurt me in the long run?

A: No, it will not. What I have discovered is that you can develop a resistance to the magnetic therapy. I often take my magnets off for a couple of days and then put them back on.

Q: How will I know it is working?

A: Like I said earlier, you may begin to take less medications. Maybe you only are taking four acetaminophen a day for your pain rather than 12. Maybe you sleep better or even only wake up twice in the night rather than every hour. Maybe you just have a little bit more energy and find you can do things that you haven't been able to do before. One easy way to know if it is working or not is to stop using it and see if your discomfort or symptoms come back. This is a sure test!

Q: Does magnetic therapy interact with any medications I am taking?

A: No, there are no drug interactions. However, I have known many people who had their medications decreased because of the benefits they had with the magnets. One person who was diabetic had more energy and began to walk more; she eventually was able to decrease her diabetic medication. This has also been reported with persons who use antihypertensives.

Q: Are you certified or licensed in magnetic therapy?

A: No, I am not. Be careful who you purchase magnets from and where you buy them. You should have someone you can discuss the use of the magnets with, as well as answer your questions.

Q: How long did you go to school to do this?

A: There is no formal education required for this. As a health care provider, I made sure and read and learned everything I could, but this was not required. I did it because I have my own standards that I practice. I would never want to tell anyone to try something unless I used it myself and I believed it could work.

Q: How can I identify a good magnet used for health care?

A: This is a very difficult question to answer. The quality of a magnet depends on its pattern and purpose for use. Since there are no FDA regulations, patients can purchase magnets of poor quality and inadequate strength and may receive no education as to their uses and side effects. You should ask around and look on the Internet for possible companies to buy from. If you purchase a magnet, you need to understand its strength. You may need a magnet with more or less gauss to be effective in providing relief for your healthcare problems. I personally would want to buy from someone who I could talk to personally and get advice from. Some tips on buying magnets include

1. Know what type of magnet you are buying. What is the strength of the gauss? Ask detailed questions.
2. Know who you are buying from. Examine the company and their reputation.
   a. Refer to the Better Business Bureau.
   b. Find out who rates the quality of their products.
3. Be aware of your payment options.
   a. Do not pay cash; credit cards offer more protection if there is a problem.
4. Be aware of your rights.
   a. Products purchased outside of the United States are not protected by the same consumer laws as products bought domestically.

Suggested Readings

Becker RO, Seldon G, Guarnaschelli MD, eds. *The Body Electric: Electromagnetism and the Foundation of Life.* New York: William Morrow & Co; 1987.

Jerabek J, Pawluk W. *Magnetic Therapy in Eastern Europe: A Review of 30 years of Research.* ISBN: 0996422708. Pawlu.

Null G. *Healing with Magnets.* New York, NY: Carroll and Graf Publishers Incorporated; 1990.

Rinker F. *The Invisible Force: Traditional Magnetic Therapy.* Ontario, Canada: Mason Service Publishing; 1997.

Vegari G. *Magnetic Therapy.* London: Caxton Editions; 2004.

Whitaker JM, Adderly B. *The Pain Relief Breakthrough: The Power of Magnets.* Boston & New York: Little, Brown, Inc; 1998.

References

1. Cuellar NG. Magnet therapy for health: a case study. Online Continuing Education Program, Honor Society of Nursing. Available at: www.nursingsociety.org/ education/case_studies/cases/SK0001.html. Accessed December 8, 2005.

2. Winemiller MH, Billow RG, Laskowski ER, Harmsen WS. Effect of magnetic vs sham-magnetic insoles on plantar heel pain: a randomized controlled trial. *JAMA.* 2003;290(11):1474–1478.

3. Rao JK, Mihaliak K, Kroenke K, Bradley J, Tierney WM, Weinberger M. Use of complementary therapies for arthritis among patients of rheumatologists. *Ann Intern Med.* 1999;131(6):409–416.

23

Reflexology

Kevin Kunz, BA

About the Author

Kevin Kunz is the president of Reflexology Research Project in Albuquerque, New Mexico. He is a reflexologist and coauthor of eight books on reflexology in 16 languages. Mr. Kunz also maintains an active website available at **www.reflexology-research.com** with several thousand hits a day.

Q: What got you interested in reflexology?

A: I picked a book off a bookstore shelf and thought it looked interesting. I tried it out on myself first and immediately fell asleep. This was unusual to me because at that time I could not fall asleep in the middle of the day. I tried my crude efforts out on family and friends. They seemed to like it and asked for more. The list grew until I was being asked to work on people outside this circle. I was prompted to learn even more about reflexology after a friend was in a head-on collision that left her partially paralyzed. That is when I decided to go into training at the National Institute of Reflexology.

I eventually began seeing many patients, working up to a 40 hour week in my practice. Many people who came to see me complained of musculoskeletal problems. However, the two most notable conditions that I treat were emphysema and paralysis. I know it was word of mouth that brought these people to me, but it was interesting that my lessons evolved around learning the capabilities of reflexology with these disorders.

I was surprised to see how reflexology impacted the outcomes of emphysema by increasing lung capacity. To my astonishment, I witnessed how one woman went from being bedridden to going back to work at a restaurant.

Q: What made you continue to pursue reflexology as a healthcare option?

A: Empirically I saw results with problems, like paralysis, that the medical profession was not able to solve. But belief alone did not do it. I needed to find out why and how reflexology was working so I began to look for the logical construct behind the practice. The most compelling case I ever had was Mrs. . who had senile dementia and did not always welcome help. One day when I was working on her husband she stopped breathing in the next room. My wife and I started CPR with no revival. My wife said, "Do what you know." I began doing reflexology, directed toward the pituitary area on her foot, a tradition revival point in reflexology. She came back immediately and started kicking. I asked Mrs. W if she knew who I was and she said, "Yes, you are a jackass." We knew she was back because she always talked like that. The ambulance had gotten lost and showed up several minutes later.

I was amazed at the quickness of her response so I researched the connection and found that the longest nerve in the body is a primary neuron running from the big toe into the brainstem. Not only was it jump starting a metabolic response, but it also was triggering what may have been a walking response. What I had thought was kicking actually looked like walking.

This incident, coupled with our experiences with paralysis, convinced us that reflexology works within the nervous system. When you apply pressure to the feet a well defined message is relayed to the brain providing feedback. The brain then adjusts the feed forward to adjust not only the muscle spindles, but also the autonomic nervous system. We were seeing this mechanism without the inhibition normally present.

Q: Does reflexology work?

A: Nothing works 100% of the time, but reflexology is so high it has kept my interest for over 25 years. I am more interested when it doesn't work.

I feel like the blind man investigating the elephant. Most people in the medical world look at reflexology as though it is some kind of outside phenomena and not the natural workings of the body. Every footstep we take involves this interaction. My wife calls reflexology weightless jogging. It is stimulating the pressure sensors in the feet without the weight bearing. It triggers changes in the autonomic nervous system (ANS) without the stress of being upright. Reports on the physiological bases of reflexology, as well as the theories for the mechanism of action, were recently published.[1]

Q: How does it work?

A: There are specific pressure points in the feet that affect every part of the body (see **Figure 23.1**). A detailed example of the map of reflex areas on the foot is available at **http://uk.dk.com/static/cs/uk/11/features/reflexology/ extract.html**.

Reflexology works by tapping into the nervous system through the proprioceptive network. Stimulating the proprioceptors does the following:

- Introduces a new signal (feedback) into the ANS causing a change in the feed forward messages coming from the brain. The new message causes a return to a more normalized homeostatic level.
- Releases endorphins which acts on free radicals. This explains the euphoric feelings a person will get from a reflexology session. This feeling of euphoria is almost universal. The exceptions usually are people with serious problems. It also explains the healing process that occurs. Lessening free radicals has been shown in Chinese research explaining why reflexology works with a wide range of complaints.

Q: How many people use reflexology?

A: Millions of people use reflexology worldwide. A more pertinent question might be how many people rub their feet when they get a headache. There are self discoverers who have found that rubbing their feet or hands will relieve various problems. This points to an arch structure existing in the nervous system that prompts this behavior.

This country is one of the few blind to the benefits of reflexology. China, Japan, and most of Europe see it as a powerful ally in working with people's health. Governments overseas are now funding studies as a public health initiative.

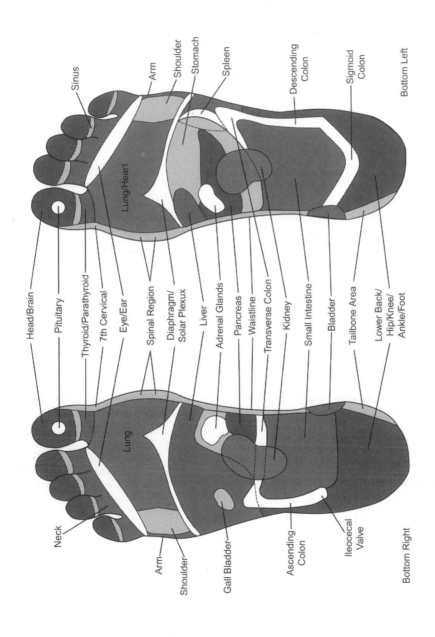

Figure 23.1   Foot Reflexology Chart

Source: Reprinted with permission from the Reflexology Research Project.

Q: What type of research has been done in reflexology?

A: Everything from randomized double-blinded controlled studies to population studies done by the government. Stephenson, Dalton, and Carlson[2] found that foot reflexology improved pain relief in cancer patients. There is an Austrian study showing a foot to body link involving the kidneys. In Ipoh, Malaysia, reflexology was used with diabetics in a public primary care clinic with over half of their patients reporting a decrease in foot pain.[3] Reflexology was shown to alleviate sensory and urinary symptoms in persons with multiple sclerosis.[4] A systemic review of pain management using reflexology was published by Stephenson and Dalton in 2003.[5]

The Chinese are measuring free radicals via blood tests that demonstrate shifts in free radicals. There are literally hundreds of studies. There are very high quality studies done to National Institutes of Health (NIH) standards on Medline. While we recognized the double blind studies as the gold standard, there are many studies that are quite fascinating.

Q: How much does reflexology cost?

A: It depends on whether it is a luxury service or a service done for say senior citizens. The average fee is about $50. A luxury service can cost over $100. I have one businessman who pays me $200 a session for being there when he needs me.

Q: Does insurance reimburse you for it?

A: I have been compensated in auto cases but the reimbursements aren't there yet for reflexology. In general it is a lost cause to try to get compensated although that does seem to be changing. There are now more reimbursements related to complementary and alternative practices.

Q: Are there any consequences to my health?

A: Reflexology is a positive stressor. With certain conditions, if done too hard, too long, and too frequently, it can become a negative stressor. In general it is very safe. The following situations require caution with reflexology: recent surgical removal of a malignant tumor; foot wounds and burns; infections or contagious diseases (e.g., scabies, common cold); unstable mental conditions; unstable pregnancy (this is a litigation danger); and danger of compromising medical treatments (e.g., a treatment given during a 24 hour holter monitoring [EKG]).

Q: How do I know if the reflexology is working and not something else I am doing?

A: We aren't working in a laboratory so it is never certain. Because of my clientele, I know that there are many therapies they are pursuing. But most tell me they have noticed a change. Mostly they have started the other therapies at other times so they feel it is the reflexology. This of course is not very scientific, but it is strong enough to keep a client coming back for treatment.

This is why research examining the outcomes of reflexology is so critical. Frequently during a reflexology session, clients have to go to the bathroom. I was very impressed when I discovered a clinical trial study (double-blinded) that demonstrated a change in arterial blood flow to the kidneys with reflexology using a kidney Doppler sonogram. It made sense of the sudden dashes I have experienced for my clients from the very earliest days of my practice.

In general however, people just know they are getting better. The businessman I mentioned earlier once said that when he goes to the doctor he gets some pills or whatever and he doesn't know if he will get better. When he sees me he feels better right away. That is what he is paying for. He sees the doctor for his concerns. He sees me to get that feeling of well being.

Q: What will my doctor think about this?

A: I used to do what I called "undercover work" in hospitals to avoid prosecution. Now I can work in the open. Although I am still called a quack and ridiculed by a lot of doctors, there is a change. Reflexologists are no longer being thrown in jail. That is a step forward.

In 1970 there was an attempt to stop a reflexology book from being published by Prentice Hall. The author was threatened with jail. I have been threatened with jail for my views. That has stopped. Now it is just name calling. But things have changed. I was working on my nephew who had flesh-eating bacteria. The doctor examining him turned to me and told me to be sure to (sic) "work on the lungs." That was the day I moved from the back of the bus to the front.

Q: Do I need to approve reflexology with my doctor before I start using it?

A: It would be great to have that kind of open communication, but I find most of my clients won't tell their doctors because of fear of ridicule. It reminds me of the warning to see your doctor before starting any exercise program. Does anyone actually do that? If a person told a doctor that they were considering reflexology, what would the doctor say? Would ridicule follow? Yes, I think you should tell your doctor. I think it makes sense to have that knowledge in order to be aware of factors influencing the patient's health. I always encourage it.

Q: Will reflexology hurt me in the long run?

A: Reflexology is a natural thing. We have had a debate within the profession for years over working on pregnant women. I think it is an urban myth and encourage research in the area. I don't think of pregnant women as being ill. Rather I think again of reflexology being a positive stressor and that if a woman has an unstable pregnancy, caution should be taken.

In the long run I think that the feet contribute step by step to our health. I have not only seen lives saved with reflexology, but lives improved with reflexology. I have also seen more pleasant deaths.

I think only research will clear this up. I think of reflexology as an exercise and just like exercise you should avoid overdoing it. Never let anyone push past your comfort zone. Report any unusual happenings to your reflexologist and your doctor.

Q: How will I know it is working?

A: I ask the client how they feel after a session. Most reply that they feel relaxed. The ones that don't are an uphill battle. For the ones that do feel relaxed, I ask them how long the relaxation effect lasts. That is the gauge on whether it is working. The relaxation response allows your body to go into a state of self-repair. If you are feeling relaxed, the reflexology is working.

Q: Does reflexology interact with any medications I am taking?

A: With the exception of insulin, I would say not to my knowledge. In fact, with insulin there is a study that found reflexology helps with insulin absorption, so the diabetic should be more closely monitored as adjustments in medications may have to be monitored.

Q: Are you certified or licensed in what you do?

A: Yes, I am certified through a private concern. No, I am not licensed since this only exists in North Dakota. The process I went through was simple. You went to a weekend class and the next year took the test. Now it is a little more complex but still lacking the necessary elements to get true respect from the medical profession. One example of an educational program is the International College of Universal Reflexologies that provides a reflexology certification program for licensed massage therapists. More information on this program is available at **www.reflexologyschools.com/index.html**.

On the other side of the coin, reflexology is a perfectly evolved, low-cost healthcare system. The simplicity of the education process makes reflexology accessible to a wide range of people. As reflexology gets more recognized, I am afraid that regulation may eliminate this low cost healthcare system. We have already seen the destructive consequences of massage regulation on reflexology.

Once massage therapy became a recognized profession in many states, massage laws were used to monopolize many of the other Complementary and Alternative Medicine (CAM) fields, including reflexology. In states like New York and Florida, you only need a massage license and no formal training is required in reflexology, Feldenkrais, or Rolfing. We call them super licenses because the states have fully qualified these license holders to practice over 200 CAM practices without any sort of training. Since reflexology may be considered a form of massage therapy, I have compiled a list of city and state requirements for the practice of reflexology, which is available at **www.reflexology-research.com/LAWS_1.html**.

This has left the efforts of professionalization difficult at best. It is hard to get certification if you can't legally practice in the first place. I can't practice in New York, Florida, and several other states. I might be arrested and in some cases charged with a felony. My wife and I were put out of business in the city of Albuquerque because of a similar law. To qualify we would have had to take training in our own book from the local massage school. Since our first book, *Complete Guide to Foot Reflexology*, was considered a standard text in reflexology, this was the case in many areas.

Licensing because of these laws has been slow. But several states and cities have recognized these problems. Texas and San Diego when confronted with the facts, changed their regulations. North Dakota has the first licensing law. Tennessee has enacted a law to recognize reflexology. The outcome of these ordinances is evident. Instead of getting reflexology in the American traditional way, you now get a foot massage instead. Untrained and undertrained practitioners, a product of the massage school growth, have hurt our reputation.

Q: How long did you go to school to do this?

A: Actually, it used to be taught in weekend seminars. Now there are courses of 200 hours or more. The Reflexology Association of America has identified a list of schools for reflexology available at: **www.reflexology-usa.org/ reflexology_schools.htm**.

Technique is taught in many courses that include pressure using the thumb, fingers, and hand. Some teach theory, but most do not. Assessment has come to the forefront as the newest addition to course work. It includes what we call reading the feet or looking for stress cues in the feet.

Since we have been so estranged from the medical system, only now are we seeing the addition of anatomy and physiology formally in course work. For example, before you learned what the pancreas did in order to understand why you worked on it. This interplay was important for the lay practitioners learning reflexology. While it is important to work the whole foot, it is also important that the areas you emphasize focus on the individual's condition. Of course you had to be careful not to diagnosis, prescribe, or treat for a specific disorder. Otherwise you were in legal trouble. So training used to be an odd mix of how to treat for a specific disorder while disclaiming actually doing it. Today it is a little better, but far from perfect.

Q: Are there standards in choosing a reflexologist to work with? How can I find a good reflexologist?

A: Traditional reflexology has standards such as good technique application, but because reflexology is an archetype there are many approaches. Some are more acupressure-like to an almost meditative quality of the Metamorphic technique. The traditional American technique had three basic pressure techniques of thumb walking, finger walking, and hook and back up. A good reflexologist applies pressure effectively within the client's comfort zone. The reflexologist should be able to vary their technique to accommodate the individual.

I think the most important outcome of the reflexology session is that you have a relaxation response, a keystone of any reflexology session. Although a foot massage is relaxing, the profound relaxation response of a reflexology session is legendary. It is this deep relaxation that allows the body to repair itself and probably accounts for the "miracles" commonly attributed to reflexology.

Suggested Readings

Kunz B, Kunz K. *Complete Guide to Foot Reflexology.* Alberquerque, NM: Reflexology Research Project; 2005.

Kunz K, Kunz B. (1992). *Hand and Foot Reflexology: A Self Help Guide.* 2nd ed. New York, NY: Simon & Schuster; 1992.

Kunz K, Kunz B. *Hand Reflexology Workbook.* 2nd ed. Alberquerque, NM: Reflexology Research Project

Kunz K, Kunz B. *Medical Applications of Reflexology, Findings in Research about Safety, Efficacy, Mechanism of Action and Cost Effectiveness of Reflexology.* Alberquerque, NM: Reflexology Research Project; 1999.

Kunz, K. & Kunz, B. *My Reflexologist Says Feet Don't Lie.* Alberquerque, NM: Reflexology Research Project; 2001.

Reflexology Research Project Presents. Available at: www.reflexology-research.com

Foot Reflexologist. Available at: www.foot-reflexologist.com

My Reflexologist. Available at: www.myreflexologist.com

References

1. Tiran D, Chummun H. The physiological basis of reflexology and its use as a potential diagnostic tool. *Complement Ther Clin Pract.* 2005;11(1):58–64.

2. Stephenson N, Dalton JA, Carlson J. The effect of foot reflexology on pain in patients with metastatic cancer. *Applied Nursing Research.* Nov 2003;16(4):284–286.

3. Remli R, Chan SC. Use of complementary medicine amongst diabetic patients in a public primary care clinic in Ipoh. *Med J Malaysia.* 2003;58(5):688–693.

4. Siev-Ner I, Gamus D, Lerner-Geva L, Achiron A. Reflexology treatment relieves symptoms of multiple sclerosis: a randomized controlled study. *Mult Scler.* 2003;9(4):356–361.

5. Stephenson NL, Dalton JA. Using reflexology for pain management: a review. *J Holistic Nurs.* 2003;21(2):179–191.

24

Research in Complementary and Alternative Medicine

Edzard Ernst, PhD, MD, FRCP(Edin.)

About the Author

Edzard Ernst is a physician in Germany where he also completed his PhD theses. He was professor in Physical Medicine and Rehabilitation (PMR) at Hannover Medical School (Germany) and head of the PMR Department at the University of Vienna (Austria). He came to the University of Exeter in 1993 to establish the first Chair in Complementary Medicine. He is founder and editor-in-chief of two medical journals (*FACT* [*Focus on Alternative and Complementary Therapies*] and *Perfusion*). His work has been awarded with nine scientific prizes and awards. He serves on the Medicines Commission of the British Medicines and Healthcare Products Regulatory Agency and on the Scientific Committee on Herbal Medicinal Products of the Irish Medicines Board.

Q: What got you interested in Complementary and Alternative Medicine (CAM)?

A: Our family doctor was a world famous homoeopath. This began my interest in CAM. Later, during my medical studies, I took courses in acupuncture, autogenic training, and other modalities. After graduation from medical school, I worked in a homoeopathic hospital in Munich. Later I received training as a basic scientist and eventually ventured back into clinical medicine. During this time, CAM research became a hobby of mine, not knowing that one day it would take me over full time.

Q: How have you seen research in CAM change over the last 10 years?

A: When I was appointed in 1993 as the first Chair in Complementary Medicine, science and CAM were a bit like fire and water. From the start, I made it quite clear that I would use my science background and apply it the best I could to conduct CAM research. The United Kingdom CAM world was a bit upset. Some people felt that this meant throwing out the baby with the bathwater. Today the United Kingdom scene has changed immensely. I think even the most evangelic believers in CAM now feel that rigorous research is necessary. They may still not like it, and many still don't understand it, but they now mostly agree that simply convincing the convinced will lead nowhere and only good science will convince the skeptic. I am not implying that this change is all my merit, but I hope I have contributed to it a little. The same thing has occurred in the United States. In 1992, the Office of Alternative Medicine was established with a $2 million budget to fund CAM studies. It became the Center of Complementary and Alternative Medicine in 1999. In 2006 the Center will have grown to include a $122.6 million annual budget.

Q: How can we continue to improve the quality of CAM research?

A: To me that's obvious! You need professional researchers to do a professional job. Those CAM enthusiasts who want to use science to prove the worth of their therapy, and we have plenty of them about, often turn out to be useless when it comes to doing good science. The only approach is to test, not prove, whether CAM works. One small word of difference, but a whole different world of thinking! During my 10 years in this business, I have become very disillusioned with amateur scientists dabbling in CAM research. This begs the question, how do we attract career scientists into CAM? The answer is, I'm afraid, embarrassingly simple: money! Without sufficient research funds, no one can expect substantial amounts of high quality research. Investing in CAM research means training CAM investigators, expanding outreach programs, and facilitating integration and collaboration with CAM practitioners.

Q: How is research in CAM different than conventional medical research?

A: Many CAM practitioners are convinced that it is fundamentally different. It's individualized, but so is surgery. It's holistic, but so is any good primary care. It's subtle, but so is psychoanalysis. It's physical and thus cannot be blinded, but so is physiotherapy. There are, of course, some obstacles, for instance, in conducting randomized clinical trials (RCT) (e.g., classical homoeopathy which requires individualized remedies, doses, repeat visits, etc.). We have invented a new trial design for totally individualized therapies without even a common, measurable outcome variable.[1] What I am trying to say is that none of the obstacles are insurmountable. I have come to the seemingly arrogant conclusion that those who insist on differences in principle either have not understood science or they use this argument in an attempt to evade scientific testing. A well-trained CAM researcher should have basic research training with clinical expertise and an interest in a CAM modality.

Q: When you look at research in CAM, how is it different between the modalities, like energy medicine versus manipulative and body based systems versus mind-body?

A: Each of the modalities stem from a theoretical background. For example, mind-body therapies may use a psychology model to guide the science while manipulation therapies may use a model from physical therapy.

The research can vary from qualitative designs to true experimental designs, which could test an intervention in a double-blinded placebo clinical trial study. The research question should define the research tool and not the modality.[2]

Q: What type of research in CAM is needed?

A: Psychologists will doubtlessly answer psychological research, and sociologists will find sociological research most important. As a physician, I strongly insist that clinical research into efficacy and safety are of paramount relevance. Patients are helped more if we define which modality does more good than harm than if we evaluate attitudes, motives, and such things. I know that many will find this politically incorrect, but who cares? I think political correctness is a far second to the welfare of our patients.

There are many gaps in the CAM literature. We lack meta-analysis, qualitative studies, clinical trials, health services, and cost and reimbursement studies. We lack extensive, longitudinal studies with large sample sizes to control for variability. We lack studies on the safety and efficacy of herbs and natural products, specifically interactions with other drugs.

Q: What standard scientific research methods are used in CAM?

A: We use mostly clinical trials, both randomized as well as uncontrolled (depending on the research question), systematic reviews (including meta-analyses), and epidemiological methods such as surveys (both cross-sectional and longitudinal). I should, however, stress again that there are no intrinsically good or bad research tools in CAM or in any other research area. There are, however, a lot of bad matches between the research tool and the research question.

Q: How are the issues of research methodologies of concern like large sample sizes, randomization, etc.?

A: Sample size and randomization are two of the many study design features that are potentially important. Sample size matters, for instance, in clinical trials. If such a study is too small it may generate a false negative result. Sample size depends, amongst other factors, on the size of treatment effect. In CAM this is usually small which means sample size has to be large. Large sample size, in turn, means high cost. As research money is scarce in CAM, we often face problems.

    Randomization is an important feature of controlled clinical trials. It is just about the only way to reduce selection bias, i.e., making sure that the two treatment groups in a typical controlled trial are comparable. If they are not, any difference at the end of the study may look as though it was produced by the therapy under scrutiny, but in fact, it could be due to selection bias. The bottom line is that nonrandomized trials can easily produce misleading results.

Q: What type of CAM studies are needed in relation to public health like social, cultural, political, and economic issues related to CAM, as well as health disparities?

A: In my view, public health depends foremost on the efficacy and safety of the modalities. Thus we need more than anything else, RCTs and prospective safety studies along the lines of post-marketing surveillance studies. All other research issues are, in my opinion, secondary. I know, social scientists and others at the "soft" end of CAM research would like to lynch me for this statement, yet I still think it's correct.

Q: How is CAM research prioritized?

A: Once it's clear that safety and efficacy are priorities, we need to ask, of which modalities? Our strategy in this respect was to not ride hobby horses but to focus on those modalities which are the most popular in your country. Finally, if this, for instance, means studying the efficacy and safety for acupuncture, we need to define for which conditions. Again this seems quite straight forward to me. I would focus on those conditions acupuncture is mostly used for, and if this leaves me several options I would opt for the one that is most important in terms of human suffering or societal costs.[3]

Research priorities, after safety and efficacy, involve: how many people use a certain modality; how much is being spent on the modality; the expense of the modality. In other words, is the public spending a lot of money on something that may not be safe and efficacious? An example of this is glucosamine. Five years ago everyone was spending money on this product, but we didn't know for sure if it worked or not. Now, we have the research to back up its efficacy.

Q: How can CAM be standardized to develop specific protocols for design validity (i.e., spirituality, bioelectromagnetic therapy, art therapy, hypnosis, meditation)?

A: This can be a tricky one. As scientists, we ideally want to standardize interventions. Complementary and Alternative Medicine practitioners often insist that they need to individualize for their approach to work. Take, for instance, homoeopathy. Depending on the precise situation, it could be silly from the homoeopaths' view to standardize therapy for a trial. This would, in their view, already predetermine a negative result. The solution is to understand these issues and design the trial such that all interest groups and experts are happy with it. One sometimes needs a bit of innovative thinking, but usually can find solutions that work. The important point here is that if individualization is required, it can be quite easily incorporated in a rigorous RCT which is still reproducible.[4] Reproducibility is crucial; there is no value whatsoever in doing irreproducible CAM research.

Q: How can we invest in high quality research in CAM? How is this done?

A: Funding for CAM research is very difficult. The dilemma is that we are often faced with the following vicious cycle: we do not have enough preliminary data to develop sound hypotheses, therefore we don't get funding to do research, and therefore we don't generate enough preliminary data to develop hypotheses.[5] To break the cycle, I think professional CAM organizations and private organizations should step in by setting aside adequate funds for research (e.g., from their membership fees). If the CAM world does not demonstrate this level of commitment, how can we expect major funders to become convinced that CAM research is a priority?

In the Unites States, NCCAM (NIH) funds research. There are no funding grants for CAM from the Agency for Healthcare and Quality (AHRQ), the CDC, the VA, Medicare, or Social Security Disabilities.

Q: How are CAM investigators being trained?

A: The answer, I fear, is often badly! In the United Kingdom we have too many CAM professionals and science amateurs dabbling in research. This leads to obvious misunderstanding, such as researching to prove instead of to test efficacy.[6] My view, after many disappointments in this area during the last 10 years, is that CAM researchers need to be scientists first and CAM experts second. This strategy would have the additional bonus of eliminating some of the extremely obvious biases that so often creep into CAM research. There are not enough researchers who have been adequately trained in CAM. For this reason, it is a major priority for NCCAM. The T32s research source awards enable institutions to train CAM researchers. There are currently nine educational centers that train CAM researchers:

- University of Arizona
- Bastyr University
- Florida International University
- Harvard Medical School
- Minnesota Consortium for CAM Clinical Research
- Morgan State University
- University of Pennsylvania, School of Medicine
- University of Virginia
- Weill Medical College of Cornell University

Q: Are there outreach activities specifically for research and CAM?

A: NCCAM recognizes the importance of disseminating research findings to the public and practitioners. The center operates a clearinghouse, partnered with the National Library of Medicine, to maintain and update CAM information on PubMed. The NCCAM web site also provides information and resources for the consumer, practitioner, and researcher.

Q: What ethical concerns are related to research and CAM?

A: Ethical concerns are the same as in conventional medicine.[7,8] They are perhaps more acute in CAM because, unlike conventional physicians, CAM providers may not have had a thorough education in medical ethics. Thus their understanding of ethical issues may not be sufficiently developed. For instance, I wonder whether the typical chiropractor, before treating a patient suffering from neck pain with cervical manipulation, obtains full informed consent that includes the following aspects:

- Neck pain does not usually require urgent treatment.
- Manipulation is not of proven efficacy for neck pain.[9]
- It may lead to severe complications in an unknown number of cases.[10]
- It leads to minor, transient adverse effects in about 50% of cases.[10]
- There are other treatments for neck pain, for example therapeutic exercises, which are probably safer and as effective.[11]

Being self-employed, most CAM providers may find it difficult to fully inform their patients in this way.[12] See Chapter 3 of this book for more information on the ethics and CAM.

Q: **What state-of-the-art clinical research is being done in CAM now?**

A: There is so much excellent research going on at present. Advances continue in identifying the mechanisms of action for the CAM modalities. There are more Phase I and II clinical trials that will answer how these modalities work, adding to the science of CAM. There are also several journals in CAM devoted to research and reporting new findings as they develop.

Q: **Can evidenced-based practice and outcomes research be utilized in CAM?**

A: I'm in danger of repeating myself: there are no bad methods only bad matches between method and question. Thus, outcomes research has its place as does any other method. While it may be difficult to determine the outcomes of so many modalities, the effects of CAM must be defined. This must be done through scientific-based instruments and measurements to match the individual CAM modality. We still have not developed adequate instrumentation to measure these outcomes.[13,14]

Q: **Drug interactions, safety and efficacy, and risks versus benefits are always issues in CAM. How have clinical investigations progressed in this area in CAM research?**

A: You can see this by an increasing number of systematic reviews of many of the modalities. Several of these publications have been mentioned in this book. For us, safety issues have always had priority.[15] We have published dozens of systematic reviews on this subject and publish a half-yearly updated report. One of the most exciting new initiatives in this area is perhaps our collaboration with the World Health Organization Monitoring Centre in Uppsala. They have on record several hundred thousand case reports of adverse events associated with herbal medicine. We are hoping to evaluate them in a scientific way.

Q: **How can we facilitate the dialogue between CAM practitioners and medical practitioners?**

A: This can be difficult. In the end, I think, we have to all realize that we are pulling on the same string. We all want the same thing: to improve future healthcare for the benefit of patients. Integrative Medicine is an attempt to do this. See Chapter 26 for more information in Integrative Medicine.

Q: **Where do you see CAM research going in the next 10 years?**

A: It will have to adopt the thinking and methods of evidence-based medicine (EBM). I think EBM is not a threat but an unprecedented chance for CAM. It also must have documented, scientific evidence on the mechanism of action seen through Phase I and II trials. Another important factor that will impact the CAM research and preparation of well-educated CAM researchers is the support of higher education (offering CAM academic and training programs in undergraduate and graduate curriculums.[16]

Q: How do you see CAM impacting health care in the next 10 years?

A: Those modalities that are evidence-based will find their way into the routine of medical practice. This hopefully will improve health care. I am also confident that CAM will lead to a re-think in conventional medicine as far as the complex but important area of the therapeutic relationship is concerned. To put it bluntly, CAM practitioners could teach physicians to become better doctors.

Suggested Readings

National Center for Complementary and Alternative Medicine (NCCAM). Available at: http://nccam.nih.gove/htdig/search.html

References

1. Ernst E. Resch K. The "optional cross-over design" for randomized controlled trials. *Fundam Clin Pharmacol.* 1995;995(9):508–511.

2. Vickers A, Cassileth B, Ernst E, et al. How should we research unconventional therapies? A report from the Conference on Complementary and Alternative Medicine Research Methodology, National Institute of Health. *Int J Technol Assess Health Care.* 1997;13:111–121.

3. Ernst E. Research priorities in CAM. *Complement Ther Med.* 2001;9(3):186–187.

4. White A, Slade P, Hunt C, Hart A, Ernst E. Individualised homeopathy as an adjunct in the treatment of childhood asthma: a randomised placebo controlled trial. *Thorax.* 2003;58:317–321.

5. Buchanan DR, White JD, O'Mara AM, Kelaghan JW, Smith WB, Minasian LM. Research-design issues in cancer-symptom-management trials using complementary and alternative medicine: lessons from the National Cancer Institute Community Clinical Oncology Program experience. *J Clin Oncol.* 2005;23(27):6682–6689.

6. Ernst E, Canter P. Investigator bias and false positive findings in medical research. *Trends in Pharmacol Sci.* 2003;24(5):219–221.

7. Caspi O, Holexa J. Lack of standards in informed consent in complementary and alternative medicine. *Complement Ther Med.* 2005;13(2):123–130.

8. Glazer J. The ethics of alternative medicine: an alternative standard? *Family Pract Manage.* 2005;12(4):13–14.

9. Ernst E. Chiropractic spinal manipulation for neck pain—a systematic review. *J Pain.* 2003;4:417–442.

10. Stevinson C, Ernst E. Risks associated with spinal manipulation. *Am J Med.* 2002;112:566–570.

11. Ernst E, Pittler M, Stevinson C, White AR. *The Desktop Guide to Complementary and Alternative Medicine.* Edinburgh: Mosby; 2001.

12. Ernst E, Cohen MH. Reply to letter by Ruhl "Spiritual informed consent for CAM." *Arch Intern Med.* 2002;162:943–944.

13. Long AF. Outcome measurement in complementary and alternative medicine: unpicking the effects. *J Altern Complement Med.* 2002;8(6):777–786.

14. Riley D, Berman B. Complementary and alternative medicine in outcomes research. *Altern Therap Health Med.* 2002;8(3):36–37.

15. Ernst E. Risks associated with complementary therapies. In: Dukes MNG, Aronson JK (eds). *Meyler's Side Effects of Drugs.* 14th ed. Amsterdam: Elsevier Science; 2000.

16. Wyatt G, Post-White J. Future direction of complementary and alternative medicine (CAM) education and research. *Semin Oncol Nurs.* 2005;21(3):215–224.

25

Integrating Clinical Practice with Complementary and Alternative Medicine

Victoria E. Slater, PhD, RN, AHN-BC

About the Author

Victoria E. Slater has a private holistic nursing practice in Clarksville, TN, where she uses a variety of CAM modalities to help people become healthier in body, mind, emotions, and spirit. Throughout her 36-year nursing career, she has taught nursing and worked on medical-surgical nursing floors, specialized in rheumatology and oncology nursing, and currently specializes in energetic therapies. Her doctoral dissertation was the first study on the effect of Healing Touch on pain.

Q: What got you interested in Complementary and Alternative Medicine (CAM)?

A: I became interested in CAM after being a cancer nurse specialist and a hospice nurse for a number of years. When I was a hospital nurse, I didn't have much of a concept of holism. I was more comfortable with the usual nursing routine and caring for patients. When I moved to hospice, I realized that the person's body was not the key to healing, but the entire situation was, including family, emotions, thoughts, and the meaning the illness had for the person. That was when holism started to make sense to me. A holistic nurse tries to help people change what they want to change to bring more balance into their physical, mental, emotional, spiritual lives and into their family and environment.

As I started to realize that health and wellness was more than biological, I joined the American Holistic Nurses' Association and began to read about and meet nurses who cared for patients in a holistic manner. Not only did they attend to the usual nursing concerns, they also broached spiritual concerns. They developed themselves and their skills to be able to care for the person more fully, more holistically. One way to do so is to practice a complementary therapy that addresses body, mind, emotions, and spirit. I found that in Healing Touch, a relative of Therapeutic Touch.

Q: How do you incorporate CAM into your holistic nursing clinical practice?

A: When I realized that I would find it difficult to incorporate a holistic philosophy and CAM in a traditional nursing job, I opened a free standing, private, holistic nursing practice. I currently offer Healing Touch, Reiki, Craniosacral and Bowen Therapies, Integrative Hypnotherapy, and Clinical Aromatherapy, plus 36 years of nursing experience. My nursing background gives me the ability to recognize how people are unbalanced in their bodies, in their lives, and in their efforts to take care of themselves. I select the modalities that I think will best help each person bring more wholeness into their lives, and those modalities that will help people begin to take care of themselves more holistically.

Q: Do all holistic nurses practice CAM?

A: No, many continue to work in the traditional nursing settings because that is where most of the patients seek care. Most holistic nurses blend their awareness of the wholeness and holiness of people in traditional nursing practices.

Q: Why did you choose the CAM modalities you practice?

A: I believe that the CAM modalities I practice are based upon similar laws of physics, especially electromagnetic and quantum physics. Healing Touch and Reiki create electromagnetic interactions between the client and practitioner to allow changes in the client's state. Craniosacral and Bowen Therapies use slight physical manipulation to set up electrical currents that induce electrical changes in the client's body. Those changes enable the person to release tension allowing the body to relax into a healthier, more balanced state. I use clinical aromatherapy for aromas' electromagnetic frequencies as well as for their biological properties. Aromas also assist a person to release tensions and stress. As clients release tension, they can open to their unexplored emotions, thoughts, and beliefs. To aid them, I studied Integrative Hypnotherapy, a non-traditional hypnotherapy approach, to help people process what they release, and to ensure that I do not introduce an inadvertent hypnotic suggestion during their time with me.

Q: Why do you think CAM really works?

A: Because I've experienced it myself. It was my experience with Healing Touch that convinced me that some CAM are legitimate healing modalities. I've tried many of the modalities discussed in this book as well as others not mentioned and have found all of them useful.

Q: How do you think CAM works?

A: Most CAM are physics-based modalities. We understand biology-based therapies, such as surgery and medicines, but most people have no clue about their electrical and electromagnetic nature. If physicists are correct, electrical or electromagnetic forces precede the development of cells, tissues, and organs. If the electromagnetic structure is damaged, the cells, tissues and organs will not function optimally. If we can heal the electromagnetic structure, a healthier body will result. Complementary and Alternative Medicine modalities such as acupuncture, acupressure, Reiki, Therapeutic Touch and Healing Touch, and bioelectromagnetic therapies work directly with the electromagnetic structure. Other CAM, such as art and music therapies, hypnosis, prayer, and meditation help a person address those feelings that have helped damage their electromagnetic structure, feelings such as rage and deep grief. Biofeedback, Tai Chi, and yoga can do the same if one pays attention to their responses to these experiences.

Q: Are there accessible books (or books for the non-specialist) that can help me understand the laws of modern physics?

A: Yes. A number of books on modern physics are geared to the non-physicist. Fruitjof Capra's *The Tao of Physics* and Gary Zukar's *The Dancing Wu Li Masters* are two of my favorites. I also like anything written by Fred Alan Wolf, especially *The Eagle's Quest*. Paul Davies is another of my favorite interpreters of modern physics, especially his book *The Matter Myth*, which he co-authored with John Gribbin. Nick Herbert's *Quantum Reality* does an excellent job of introducing eight separate quantum theories that nonphysicists tend to squash together. Capra puts together a number of modern scientific concepts in *The Web of Life*. Two books that explore the role of consciousness in quantum physics are Herbert's *Elemental Mind* and Wolf's *The Spiritual Universe: How Quantum Physics Proves the Existence of the Soul*. Once you have even an elemental understanding of the quantum theories, many of the CAM modalities begin to make sense.

Q: How do I know which CAM are for me?

A: This is a very good question. I would recommend you consider the following:

- Recognize your personal philosophical framework. Do you believe your body, mind, emotions, and spirit are separate or do they interact? How do you think your emotions and thoughts affect your body? If you believe that your body, mind, emotions, and spirit are separate, then you will be more comfortable with different types of CAM than someone who believes that they are integrated.
- Decide what you want to accomplish for yourself and your own health. Check out the various CAM in your area to see if they will do what you want. You may have options in your area you were not aware of.
- Decide how much control you want in your healthcare regime. Some CAM enable you to be actively involved, such as Therapeutic and Healing Touch and Integrative Hypnotherapy. In other CAM, such as acupuncture, you will be more passive. Of course, the degree of involvement you have is your choice and determined by your personal goals. The more actively involved you are in your own healing, the more rapidly you will notice changes.
- Ask friends what they have tried and what the results were. Talk to other people who may have the same goals you have for your health care. Get feedback from others; be open to a variety of possibilities.
- Experiment with different modalities. Know that all of the modalities described in this book will do something for you; you have to decide if it is what you want. On the other hand, what works for some, may not work for others. A number of things will influence how receptive you may be to a certain CAM.

Q: How do I find the practitioner for me?

A: Most cities have health food stores where you can find an alternative newsletter that will list practitioners of many modalities. Check the bulletin board at health food stores; many stores let people post their business cards and announcement of classes. Some CAM practitioners have web pages or are on Internet lists. Don't limit your search to the Internet because many good CAM practitioners don't advertise. Word of mouth is the most useful way to find a good practitioner.

Q: Once I have a list of practitioners, how do I choose one?

A: Call the practitioners you've chosen and interview them. Ask about their training, qualifications, and experiences. How much training have they had in their modality? If certification is offered in that modality, are they certified? How much experience have they had using that modality? Do they practice or have they been trained in other modalities, and how much experience have they had in other healthcare fields. Essentially, you want to know something about the breath and depth of their experiences.

Q: What should I do during a CAM treatment?

A: That depends on what you want. You can simply enjoy the therapy and receive its effects. On days you are really tired, that may be the most important thing you can do for yourself. On other days, you may want to notice the emotions and thoughts that come up during the therapy. You may realize that you need to deal with these emotions and thoughts more deliberately. You may choose to see a counselor or try one of the mind-body or energetic therapies. It is important to realize that those emotions and thoughts that come up during treatments have been stored in your tissues. Dealing with them constructively may be less painful than letting them remain within you.

Q: Complementary and Alternative Medicine can be expensive and often not covered by insurance. Are they worth it?

A: They have been for me. I am healthier and happier than when I started routinely using CAM modalities. Every person will have a different experience, but if you have not found relief with your usual medical treatments, or you want to try a different approach, you may want to give CAM a try. It is important that you realize that CAM does not work instantly. The treatments are cumulative. Imagine cleaning a very dirty house. Over time and with work you can make it sparkling. If you can repair some of the damage that time has done, you can even make it better. It takes time, effort, and dedication.

One way to get the most for your money is to take classes in CAM. In many of the classes, such as Reiki, Healing Touch, and Reflexology, you will give and receive several treatments during the class. Often the cost of the class is cheaper than receiving the same number of treatments in the teacher's office. The quality of treatments will be different, however, so don't stop seeing your certified CAM practitioner.

Q: Is CAM holistic?

A: Many of the CAM modalities are holistic, especially yoga, homeopathy, Reiki, Therapeutic and Healing Touch, and Reflexology. Because they work on body, mind, emotions, and spirit at the same time, do not limit your expectations. If you come in for physical pain relief, you may experience emotional pain relief first, or vice versa.

Just because a modality is not holistic in itself, your practitioner may be. Holistic practitioners often will blend a number of CAM and traditional modalities to create an overall holistic experience for their clients.

Q: Will I feel good after every CAM treatment?

A: No, unfortunately, you may feel worse several days after a treatment. This is called a healing crisis, but it might be more accurate to say that you are releasing tension and toxins that you have stored for years. As they come out of your tissues, you will feel bad, but as they pass out of your system, you will feel much better. Wait three to five days before deciding what the treatment did for you.

Q: Are there frameworks for CAM to guide clinical practice?

A: Yes, many frameworks guide the use of complementary and alternative modalities in clinical practice. Sometimes practitioners work within a professional framework that is developed from education and training. Physicians use a medical framework, nurses use nursing models, counselors use a psychological framework, and clergy use one that is consistent with their church's teachings. Various CAM may make sense in one framework but not in another.

At the same time, a compartmentalized framework views the body, mind, emotions, spirit, and environment as separate entities, while the holistic framework views them as integrated and interacting. A professional with a compartmentalized framework will be more restricted in their use of CAM; those with a holistic framework will be more inclusive and more likely to explore widely among CAM.

A third framework is based on modern physics, which teaches that the physical body is made up of energy. Many CAM practitioners believe that if you can intervene with the energy, you can influence the body, mind, and the emotions. CAM practices such as energy therapies, homeopathy, and acupuncture are designed to intervene at the energy level.

Q: What are the nursing frameworks that guide your clinical practice and use of CAM?

A: My use of CAM as a nurse is guided, first, by the legal scope of the nursing practice within my state of residence. As a nurse, I cannot diagnose or prescribe; that is the legal right of physicians, physician assistants, and nurse practitioners. However, nursing is not about curing diseases; it is about helping people help themselves. I have incorporated into my holistic nursing practice the mind-body interventions and energy therapies that I think will best help my clients heal and help themselves.

Numerous nursing theories help frame my view of nursing. Theories that can easily be integrated with CAM include Roy's Adaptation, Rogers' Unitary Human Beings, Newman's Health as Expanding Consciousness, Parse's Human Becoming, Watson's Human Caring, and Leininger's Transcultural Nursing (**Table 25.1**). I have been taught that nursing is about caring and that nurses should be sensitive to the client's culture and philosophy. I have learned that people grow by being listened to and that they evolve gradually and at their own speeds. I've learned to listen carefully and to use my hands skillfully to ease pain and distress. The CAM that I have incorporated into my clinical practice are a natural extension of my nursing education and experience.

Q: How can the development of taxonomies help promote the use of CAM?

A: As we develop taxonomies, for example classifications, we will have a means to gather data about the use and effects of CAM. Researchers will be able to track outcomes and help put CAM modalities on a solid scientific footing. Data gathered through the use of taxonomies will help insurance companies decide which modalities to reimburse and help people find the best CAM for them. Over time, taxonomies will help reveal both which CAM are effective, leading to their recognition in a larger treatment community, and those which are less effective, causing their use to dwindle.

Taxonomies in CAM can also be helpful in research. Like any research, CAM research always requires scientific rigor and reliability and all modalities should be carefully examined. Research in the physics based CAM modalities, such as Healing Touch and other energy therapies, will require an adjustment to standard research methodology. Because energy therapies bring people into balance, research designs must take that into account. A study using healthy volunteers who are already in balance will not be an effective test of a modality that brings people into balance. Similarly, many times shams or mock therapies cannot be used in research because the human-to-human interaction that is part of energy therapies will influence the results. Research of energy therapies must involve sick people with real problems receiving treatments from trained and experienced therapists (see Chapter 24 on CAM research).

Q: How can you research CAM in a holistic nursing clinical setting?

A: Holistic nurses believe that everything about a person is connected. Research must take this into account. The client, practitioner, and treatment are interrelated, so each must be studied in a research project. The client's emotions, thoughts, medical history and CAM history, their family support, and their degree of involvement in the treatment must be taken into consideration. The practitioners' training and experience, as well as how often they give treatments, will influence results.

Table 25.1   Nursing Models that Can Be Integrated in CAM

Sister Callista Roy[1]	Roy Adaptation Model	"Adaptation Model" says we are adaptive, our environment is an internal and external stimulus and health is a part of becoming whole in the adaptive environment. This adaptation includes spirituality. Matter and energy are a part of organization that includes self-organization, consciousness, awareness, creativity, thinking and feeling, transformation, and integration with human and environment needed to adapt.
Martha Rogers[2]	Science of Unitary Beings	"Unitary Human Beings" all have "energy" with openness that is exchanged and integral to our environment.
Margaret Newman[3]	Health as Expanding Consciousness	"Expanding Consciousness" is becoming more of oneself, finding a greater meaning of life, and connecting with other people. There is a "Universal Force" that connects all things. Humans are open energy systems. The consciousness is how the person interacts with the environment. Everything is related to movement–space–time.
Rosemarie Parse[4]	Human Becoming	"Human Becoming" is a spiritual approach that examines quality of life and value of life. It involves living in the moment—trascendence or moving beyond the "now" in the midst of ambiguity and change.
Jean Watson[5]	Caring Theory	"Caring" includes carative factors like hope, trust, and expression; also includes emerging concepts like transpersonal mind–body spirit, consciousness to promote healing, and consciousness as energy and wholeness.
Madeline Leinenger[6]	Transcultural Theory	"Caring" is the essence of nursing and includes knowledge of generic, folk, and indigenous ways of caring that varies in different cultures. Nursing care is specific to Folk Systems (folk medicine). Holistic Health and Well Being is influenced by religion, kinship, society, culture, values, economic, and education.

Q: How do you work with other members of a healthcare team to coordinate a treatment plan for a patient?

A: If a client is actively seeing another healthcare provider, I ask the client if I can send a letter to that provider telling them what I am doing and the results I expect. I always tell the client what I expect to happen and explain how the CAM treatment might interact with their medical treatments.

Q: How do CAM treatments interact with medical treatments?

A: Energy work will enhance healing rates, including post-operatively. Cancer patients who are receiving chemotherapy may not be as sick or tired after their therapy. Oncologists need to know that the patient is receiving energy therapies because some chemotherapy dosages are adjusted according to the patient's toxic reactions. Patients who don't get very sick after chemotherapy because they are receiving energy therapies may get too strong a chemotherapy dose.

Numerous medications may need to be adjusted for a patient who is receiving CAM treatments. For example, massage and energy therapies may gradually decrease blood pressure, which may require the physician to lower blood pressure medicine dosages. Some CAM modalities may decrease depression, reducing the person's need for antidepressants. Be sure to ask your CAM practitioner how the treatment may interact with your other therapies.

Q: How do you empower other members of the healthcare profession to buy into CAM?

A: I don't try. People must be true to themselves. If someone is not willing to investigate or try CAM, I cannot change their minds. Effective CAM will stand the test of time. I believe that as more and more people experience CAM and are happy with the results the healthcare system will change on its own accord.

Suggested Readings

American Holistic Nurses Association. Available at: *www.ahna.org*

Healing Touch. Available at: *www.healingtouch.net*

Capra F. *The Tao of Physics.* Boston, MA: Random House; 1999.

Zukav G. *The Dancing Wu Li Masters.* New York, NY: William Morrow & Co; 1979.

Wolf F. *The Eagle's Quest.* New York, NY: Touchstone; 1991.

Davies P, Gribbin, J. *The Matter of Myth.* New York, NY: Simon & Schuster; 1992.

Herbert N. *Quantum Reality.* New York, NY: Random House; 1992.

Capra F. *The Web of Life.* New York, NY: Random House; 1996.

Herbert N. *Elemental Mind.* New York, NY: Plume Publishers; 1994.

Wolf F. *The Spiritual Universe.* Portsmouth, NH: Moment Point Press, Inc; 1998.

References

1. Roy C. Andrews H. *The Roy Adaptation Model.* 2nd ed. Stamford, CT: Appleton & Lange; 1999.
2. Rogers M. *The Science of Unitary Human Beings.* Thousand Oaks, CA; 1991.
3. Newman M. *Health as Expanding Consciousness.* 2nd ed. New York, NY: Harry Abrams; 1994.
4. Parse R. *Theory of Health as Human Becoming.* Thousand Oaks, CA: Sage Publications; 1992.
5. Watson, J. *Nursing: Human Science and Human Care: A Theory of Nursing.* Sudbury, MA: Jones and Bartlett; 1999.
6. Leininger M, McFarland M. *Transcultural Nursing.* 3rd ed. New York, NY: McGraw-Hill; 2002.

26

Integrative Medicine:
The Common Ground?

David Reilly, FRCP, MRCGP, FFHom

About the Author

David Reilly is the director of the Centre for Integrative Care at the Glasgow Homeopathic Hospital in Glasgow, Scotland.

Q: What got you interested in Integrative Medicine?

A: I am a doctor who has studied a number of approaches to patient care. I have come to the conclusion that the quality of our vision in health care will determine the future. So I offer some thoughts on what might be useful for healthcare providers to aim for, and discuss some values to aspire to. I will also discuss where we in modern medicine are now, consider how we got there, and wonder how we might go forward to integrate Complementary and Alternative Medicine (CAM) in health care.

Q: How do you see the future in CAM and conventional medicine?

A: Let us first consider what unites us more than what divides us, whatever our type of practice: conventional, complementary, or alternative. I suggest we build bridges between us by considering a shared study of healing and healing responses, a common ground.

Imagine a room with multiple doors and windows. We enter through our portal, it is labelled as we are: conventional, CAM, acupuncturist, doctor, nurse, counsellor, or any healthcare provider. As we sit down, we are surprised to find that we are sitting with anthropologists, spiritual carers, artists, story tellers, biologists, historians, or any other discipline with something to teach about creative change and building a better life.

We sit around a large circular table. We are asked to consider the space in the middle of the table. We are encouraged to speak of the common ground that unites us. We are asked in one sense to leave our discipline at the door. If we mention it, it is to be only in the context of what it has taught us about this common ground, and even more challengingly, we have to express this in ordinary shared terms, accessible to all.

Q: What would be the focus of this interdisciplinary group?

A: The common ground is our communal humanity. Our shared desire is caring for others and bringing about creative change for those who are suffering in some way.

Too often our disciplines, and so our discussions, divide us. We can even identify who we are by our technical skills. Yet, in truth, our discipline and technical skills are the vehicles we use to express the reason we went into caring work. We all want to make a difference in people's lives and experiences.

Q: How do you think this discussion would evolve?

A: Led by the historian, we begin to discuss our tribal tendencies, our war modes, our arrogance, and our drive to prove our approach is the best and most prestigous. We are reminded of our capacity for quackery and foolishness and fashion. Then the anthropologist tells us how each and every human tribe is united by the curious fact that when a person is vulnerable they might seek the help of a specialist. This specialist will listen, understand, and reflect back to us in new, more healing ways. Together the parties in this alliance build a symbolic bridge between them. Through rituals and symbols, a new understanding of what is needed is understood. But always—be it with chicken bones, needles, drugs, aromatherapy, prayer, touch, etc.—shared intention, hope, expectation, and human ministration are given and received. The specialist provides a healing journey with identifiable stages marked by changing needs at every stage of the process.

Q: How would the other members of the group respond to this?

A: As everyone hears this, of course, the resonances in each work is seen, yet our focus is on enriching the common ground, not showing how sharp each discipline's chisel is. Someone else mentions that Western medicine has buried these thoughts under the idea of placebo. A social scientist quotes surveys of people's partial loss of faith in conventional medicine and their seeking of alternatives elsewhere for these shared and needed human elements.

From the dialogue, the proposal emerges that if we directly study the common ground of human caring and human healing together, we could share our experience usefully. We realize we are all humans who care about caring for others.

Seen this way it is obvious that the vision of integrating CAM and Orthodox Medicine (OM) might be a useful step, but it falls very short of where we could go. Just adding a lot more doors to the corridors of care might expand choice, but it will never in itself ensure the things we seek like clarity, integrity, safety, effectiveness, holism. So "What will achieve these things?" may be our real question.

Q: What is the goal of Integrative Care or Medicine?

A: The goal would be to achieve and demonstrate this increased coherence and decreased fragmentation in health care. Healing, growth, and a movement to wholeness are what is being sought for the patient. Paradoxically, while cure can, and mostly does, add to a person's coherence, their sense of wholeness—the underlying debate, brought out by CAM—is that too often this is achieved at the cost of a feeling of loss of personal meaning, personal integrity, and wholeness. An efficient system can still dehumanize and leave us feeling less complete. We need both technical excellence and a context and engagement that is integrative for us. Studies have shown that patient's self-report outcomes improved after one month of participating in an integrative medicine clinic with sustained effects for six months follow-up.[1]

In examining cost-effectiveness, primary care physicians who used an integrative approach to patient care had improved clinical outcomes, decreased hospitalizations, decreased in-hospital days, decreased outpatient surgeries, and decreased pharmeceutical costs when compared to conventional medical practices.[2]

Thus in this definition, CAM approaches can help, but they are not essential. Orthodox Medical care can be very integrative; CAM can be very confusing and conflicting. But the cliché holds some truth that Orthodoxy excels at cure and is poor at caring, and CAM is the complementary opposite.

Q: What got us to our current position?

A: As the gap between the two sides is narrowing, the possibility of some of the real issues coming into focus is apparent. Taking a perspective over time is helpful. Maybe in 50 years or longer will see the completion of real transformation.

We have seen a movement toward integrated medicine, which seems to be the coexistence of the OM and CAM worlds. This often seems to be an issue of practitioners of different persuasions working together or individual practitioners beginning to develop additional skills. I would see this as a step forward, but to be honest, it's not really good enough. Combination medicine (CAM added to orthodox practice) is not integrative medicine.[3] Somewhere in all this we are still avoiding confronting the central and core issues of holism and of a truly integrative approach.

Q: What is the difference between holism and CAM?

A: Holism and CAM are not the same thing. There is an arrogance that I would label "more holistic than thou" which suggests that if one studies a system that takes a more mind-body approach and a systems approach, that together they will produce holism. In fact, I believe that most of our disciplines are specializations, in that they look at the individual through the tinted spectacles of that worldview. I began to explore unconventional areas to exactly get away from the formula of medicalizing individual's difficulties and then prescribing an intervention. In fact so much of CAM is exactly "the pill for every ill" and can be taken to absurdity if one is not cautious.

I believe the underlying demands for CAM reflected a progressive breakdown in the healing qualities of conventional medicine. This was also seen in Orthodox Medicine when technological advances dazzled us to a point where the human dimension was underplayed. I believe we have to have the courage to try and look 20 and 30 years ahead and ask what we really want. In 1983, I published a paper that contributed to opening up the debate.[4] As well as showing the nascent rise of CAM within OM, I expressed concern that it could be "the Emperor's new clothes." People used to move between different specialists like their cardiologist, psychologist, and pharmacist. They now might circulate between their homeopath, acupuncturist, and health food store. Maybe it is a step forward, but it is not enough.

Q: Why do we need the term "integrative care"?

A: The definition takes account of the emergence of a realization that we have been dominated in recent decades by what Roger Sperry would have characterised by left hemisphere dominance, but might have been better labelled by Betty Edwards as L mode, the aspect of us that tackles life through a reductionist, linear, single cause and effect logic. It leads us, logically, to think a great creative work can be made by concentrating on the correct chisel. R mode experiences things directly, like listening to music, giving and receiving kindness, understanding the connectivity between things. Just L mode, and we are robots (the clichéd depiction of dehumanized, reductionist orthodoxy over reliant on its interventions and tools). Just R mode, and we are lost in space without planning for our survival; the clichéd picture of vague, unscientific, and fickly dangerous CAM). Call it science versus art, cure versus care, intervention versus nurturing, CAM versus Orthodox, reductionist versus holism, we still need to learn to better synthesize these and use our right and left hand together in care.

By side stepping this and looking directly at the conditions that modify healing responses, we arrive at the impact of our humanity as well as our interventions restoring our humanity and compassion to meld with our technical skills.

Q: Where are we today in achieving a concept of Integrative Care?

A: All over the world the debate is moving on from arguments based around specific CAMs; the old stark defiance of any value in CAM is countered by the overstated and under-researched counter claims. The talk is of integrative approaches, which consists of whole systems involving a relationship between the patient and the healthcare provider, multiple approaches to treatment that are both orthodox and CAM, along with the main concept of care as the intention.[3] Often that involves dialogue around the systems and models of care that are emerging and likely we need all these and more. But critically, each of these models might be integrative or fragmentary at different times for different people. We could call these parallel, serial, and integrated.

Q: Describe Models of Care versus Integrative Care?

A: The parallel model is still the most common Model of Care. Usually patient led, the patient self refers to their choice of therapist, often not telling the other therapists about this. This model can be empowering and successful. The patient knows they need a treatment and finds what is needed which may include massage, yoga, or chiropractic. Thus it can be integrative. It is supported by creating positive health outcomes, yet undermined by arrogant or isolationist attitudes by the healthcare providers.

The parallel model carries a risk of conflicting therapies, conflicting advice, and a loss of a steadying healthcare provider. It also carries a risk of fragmentation, negative interactions, and disruption. This is minimized again by enlightened attitudes on the health care providers part, encouraging the patient to allow communication between the parallel practitioners.

The serial model is a Model of Care that involves a sequential pattern. A person says, "let's see what the orthopedic doctor says, then if need be we will try chiropractic." It can have the strength of a more integrated pathway with less confusion. However, the draw back is a slower, less efficient passage relying on the level of development of the perspective and knowledge of the players involved. There could also be a power play here, either keeping patients away from what they need or capturing patients and not letting them move on.

The integrated model often involves multiple professionals. Some use a triage system, trying to select the best pathway for the client. At best, increasing the chances of being integrative, this is a loop with progress review plus contact between the healthcare providers. The healing journey is acknowledged and taken into account. Sometimes it is just a complex shopping mall model with no inherent support for integrative elements other than the important aspects of enriched choice and opportunity.

Q: Central to this are the healthcare providers in CAM. How specialized are they, and what is the scope of their training?

A: CAM providers can be specialists or generalists much like in OM. The specialist is a heat seeking missile after a narrower range of targets. That is its strength and weakness. An example of this is homeopathy. The generalist is the one who knows when the missile needs disarming and a different tactic is invoked. For the patient, the strength is not being married to any one particular discipline and having a broad perspective that helps clarify the map of the healing journey. Without this element it is hard to achieve an integrative process.

Many specialists have no understanding of the specific challenges and skills of the general practitioner (GP). A GP specializes in being a generalist and extracts primary care elements from other disciplines, such as homeopathic first aid training, to use when appropriate. The GP will refer on to a specialist when needed but continues to be the primary healthcare provider. This is used as the basis of the Glasgow Model of education that has trained around 20% of Scotland's GPs in basic homoeopathy with a subsequent pathway for those who want to go on to more specialized levels of knowledge.

There is also a special role in the community for bilingual, dual trained healthcare providers who know first hand the respective strengths and weaknesses of the different approaches (e.g., a nurse also trained in homoeopathy, a physical therapist also trained in acupuncture). The more the individual practitioner has struggled to achieve an integrative self development, the more they will pass that on. Of course some are more gifted at languages than other, and few can master more than a few. Thus risks here are of Jack-of-all-trades superficiality, but when well handled, the knowledge of such practitioners can be an invaluable contribution to the community. One way to achieve balance is to become a generalist in some dimensions and a specialist in others and have clarity about these boundaries.

Q: What are some examples of possibilities that integrative approaches yield?

A: In primary care, one approach is to take generalists, such as conventional GPs or practice nurses, and give them additional training. You can take their background knowledge and build on a discipline with specific training, giving targeted primary care extractions of the specialist model while alerting them to boundaries and the point an additional expert will be needed. For example, we have seen success with Electrostimulation Therapy incorporating Electroacupuncture for drug withdrawal and this has led to nurse run clinics. Another example is primary care homeopathic training which has been used by about 20% of Scotland's GPs (follow-up research has shown continued useful practice and results).

In specialist care the patient is guaranteed a high level consultation plus technical excellence. Direct communication flows between the specialist and the referring generalist. In Glasgow our greatest experience is with the development of a regional network of specialists. In each region of the country a patient can be referred to this doctor, who will be on the Faculty of Homoeopathy's Specialist Register.

Multidisciplinary teams involve intense case reviews with a co-ordinated team care plan. Doctors, nurses, physiotherapists, occupational therapists, massage therapists, and art therapists combine together bringing mostly dual-trained individuals plus some single discipline specialists, so that homeopathy, acupuncture, and related disciplines are combined with the full range of orthodox diagnostic and therapeutic possibilities. A key named worker, most commonly a doctor, works with the patient to ensure the whole person and integrative elements with an emphasis on self-empowerment whereever possible.

Q: Where might we go from here?

A: I have hinted at the healthy plurality of models we are all exploring. We need to advance on two fronts. One is related to techniques and tools, the other to healing.

Better Techniques: Chisels should be sharp and safe just as practitioners should be effectively trained and apply techniques well. We have a rich range of research methodologies for this, and over the next few decades we should make good progress.

Integrative Healing: The second front needs addressing in its own right. How do we achieve better integrative care? Here we need to emphasize outcome and develop new tools to capture patient experiences. In the era of evidence based medicine, how are we to reconcile this with inner personal experience? Can we get evidence based poetry? or evidence based art of medicine? This apparent absurdity is resolved if the patient's experience becomes central; people know if a poem worked for them. We need to begin to ask, and in the exploration, create a loop of feedback between research, education and practice.

Research: Research can straddle these domains and is showing some promise. We are not just having more trials, but a realization of their limits and the difficulties in producing really good, thoughtful work. To quote a character from an Arthur C. Clark novel who was designing a garden, "the laws of nature say we can only get two out of these three: quick, cheap, or good."

Q: What are some early examples of direct inquiry into the state of the art of integrative approaches?

A: I will give some examples from our work to illustrate the sort of questions we might formulate and tackle. For example, are we delivering holistic care? Was this care integrative for patients? What elements are essential to achieve an integrative effect?

System level questions: Are we delivering holistic care?

Almost 4000 GPs in Scotland were surveyed with replies from 62% (Mercer et al., 2002). Nearly 90% felt that a holistic approach was essential to providing good health care, but only 20% thought primary care was delivering it and only 6.8% thought the current organization of primary care services made it possible. The main constraint on holism within the consultation was seen as the time available, followed by the GPs own stress level. Questions and monitoring like this could help us design better care delivery systems and contexts.

Outcome of care questions: Are we delivering acceptable results?

We have used outcome studies to track patients through their care and we have been exploring new patient centered measures. For example, the Glasgow Homoeopathic Hospital Outcome Scale (GHHOS) relates outcome to the patient's judgement about impact or on the quality of daily living (**www.adhom.org**). This is the black box approach: take the baseline and measure the outcome. It says nothing about why the change occurred, but it establishes if it does. For example, we tracked 200 patients going through the integrative in-patient care program at Glasgow Homeopathic Hospital. The following results were found at a three- and six-month follow up (94% response rate):

- 70% had useful or major improvement in presenting complaint,
- 67% had useful or major improvement in general mood and well-being,
- 40% reported fewer consultations with their GP,
- 36% reported decreased use of conventional drugs,
- 33% reported fewer admissions to hospital, and
- 30% reported less outpatient or ambulatory care.

The latter cost-effectiveness data hints at an area ripe for major inquiry. Improving care questions: Was this care integrative?

To investigate patient enablement or empowerment, we used a questionnaire-based study with 200 consecutive outpatients attending four doctors at the Glasgow Homoeopathic Hospital, an National Health Service- funded integrated complementary and Orthodox medicine unit.[6] The Mean Enablement Score (using Howie's Patient Enablement Instrument) was high at 4.7, 50% higher than the average in primary care. Of the four individual doctors, the results varied with one practitioner scoring less than the others. This study points to the possibility of us beginning to monitor the level of integrative effect of our care as distinct from the medical outcome.

Q: What makes the care integrative?

A: This inquiry has begun but the results are scattered in multiple disciplines. Much work is needed. For example, we analyzed the views of the 200 patients mentioned in the previous studies. Although there were many factors that correlated with enablement, multi-regression analysis showed three key factors that accounted for 41% of the variation in enablement, with empathy being the single most important factor. These factors were patient's expectations, doctor's empathy (as perceived by the patient), and doctor's own confidence in the therapeutic relationship.

We then went on to a qualitative study to examine common themes linking the R mode discussed at the beginning of this chapter. The findings that emerged give us a solid basis for our vision of the future health care we are seeking. Patients

- valued time availability, the whole person approach, and being treated as an individual;
- felt their story was listened to for the first time and their symptoms were taken seriously;
- felt the doctors at GHH were trustworthy, compassionate, and positive, often engendering hope; and
- felt equality of relationship was a major them with a strong sense of mutual respect.[7]

Q: What is integrative change with someone? Can coherence be demonstrated?

A: Another frontier area will be our exploration of our inner space and self healing potential. Studies like those showing cardiovascular and synchronized neurological states and rhythms altering with meditation and prayer, and physiological entrainment between the patient and the carer, coupled with objective evidence for significant self-healing potential (see references) point to exciting future discoveries and promise of improved awareness of how we can better care for one another.

Suggested Reading

The Academic Departments of the Centre for Integrative Care. Available at: www.adhom.org

The American Association of Integrative Medicine. Available at: www.aaimedicine.com/main.php

The Consortium of Academic Health Centers for Integrative Medicine. Available at: www.imconsortium.org/html/membership.php

The Integrative Medicine Alliance. Available at: http://www.integrativemedalliance.org

References

1. Scherwitz LW, Cantwell M, McHenry P, Wood C, Stewart W. A descriptive analysis of an integrative medicine clinic. *J Altern Complement Med.* 2004;10(4):651–659.

2. Sarnat RL, Winterstein J. Clinical and cost outcomes of an integrative medicine IPA. *J Manipulative Physiol Ther.* 2004;27(5):336–347.

3. Bell IR, Caspi O, Schwartz GE, et al. Integrative medicine and systemic outcomes research: issues in the emergence of a new model for primary health care. *Arch Int Med.* 2002;162(2):133–140.

4. Reilly D. Young doctors' view on alternative medicine. *BMJ.* 1983;287(6388): 337–339.

5. Mercer S, Hasegawa H, Reilly D, Bikker A. Length of consultations. Time and stress are limiting holistic care in Scotland. *BMJ.* 2002;325(7374):1241.

6. Mercer S, Reilly D, Watt G. The importance of empathy in the enablement of patients attending the Glasgow Homoeopathic Hospital. *Br J Gen Pract.* 2002;52(484); 901–905.

7. diBlasi Z, Kliejnen J. Consultations at GHH. A pilot qualitative study and commentary on some therapeutic consultations. Available at: www.adhom.org/adh_download/ Consultations%20at20%20GHH.pdf Accesssed January 11, 2006.

INDEX

Page numbers followed by *t* indicate tables.

A

ACA. *See* American Chiropractic Association
Access to CAM, 29
Acupuncture and acupressure, 5, 15*t*, 36, 177–184
  Auricular Acupuncture, 179
  in combination with TCM, 58
  costs of, 181
  drug interactions, 181
  electro-acupuncture, 179
  insurance coverage for, 181
  National Certification Commission for Acupuncture and Oriental Medicine (NCCAOM), 182
  NIH support of, 14
  research on, 180–181
  risks associated with, 180
  styles of, 179
  training in, 181–182
  treatments, 179–180
  usage of, 178
Acupuncturists, 182
Acupuressure, 179. *See also* Acupuncture and acupressure
Adaptation, 252–253
Adaptation Model, 253, 254*t*
AHG. *See* American Herbalist Guild
AHMA. *See* American Holistic Medical Association
AHNA. *See* American Holistic Nurses' Association
Alaska Native traditional healing, 35, 37

Allopathic medicine, 4, 6, 7, 39
Alpha lipoic acid, 150
Alternative Health News Online, 20
Alternative medicine, 5, 10, 11*t*
Alternative therapies practitioners, 138–139
Alton, John, 185
American Association of Colleges of Nursing, 45
American Association of Integrative Medicine, 267
American Association of Naturopathic Medical Colleges, 91*t*
American Chiropractic Association (ACA) Code of Ethics, 22
American Herbalist Guild (AHG), 150
American Holistic Medical Association (AHMA), 22, 150
American Holistic Nurses' Association (AHNA), 48
  Core Curriculum, 49, 52
  Position Statement on Holistic Nursing Ethics, 23
  Standards of Advanced Holistic Nursing Practice for Graduate-Prepared Nurses, 49
  Standards of Holistic Nursing Practice, 23
American Indian Traditional healing, 37
American Journal of Acupuncture, 59
American Massage Therapy Association (AMTA), 171–172
  Code of Ethics and Standards of Practice for Massage Therapy, 172
  web site, 167, 172